A Handbook of

PRE-NATAL PAEDIATRICS

for Obstetricians and Paediatricians

A Handbook of PRE-NATAL PAEDIATRICS for Obstetricians and Paediatricians

---

Edited by

GIFFORD F. BATSTONE
M.B., B.S.
Registrar in Chemical Pathology
Bristol Royal Infirmary

ALASTAIR W. BLAIR
M.B., Ch.B., M.R.C.P.E., D.C.H.
Senior Registrar in Paediatrics
Southmead Hospital, Bristol

JACK M. SLATER
M.B., Ch.B., M.R.C.O.G.
Consultant Obstetrician
Yeovil District Hospital

MTP
Medical and Technical Publishing Co, Ltd
Aylesbury
1971

Published in the United Kingdom by
MTP
Medical and Technical Publishing Co. Ltd.
Chiltern House, Aylesbury, Bucks.

SBN 852 00032 4

First published 1971

Printed by Eyre & Spottiswoode Ltd, Thanet Press, Margate

The eye is blind to the greatest mystery
In the universe. The miniscular seed
Falling to the waiting earth of the womb,
The heat of love inadvertently sparking a
Secondary fusion, darker more basic,
Within womankind.
Womb-warmth caressing an atom of
Creation. The start of the path to daylight,
Often re-trodden – always unique.

Man holds knowledge, tabulates
Stages of growth, unravels the ingenious
Mechanics of the placenta and wonders
At creation, and wonders and wonders
And so challenges the creation of creation itself.
Will his curiosity prevail? Will he
Delve into the metaphysical realms of
Creation to explain one enigma, only to
Find himself confronted by another – even greater.

PATRICK JOHN CORCORAN

FOREWORD

Formerly the policy of masterly inactivity was generally accepted in obstetrical practice. However, this is no longer true at the beginning of the present decade, and the authors are to be congratulated in trying to stimulate their juniors to approach the problems of Pre-natal Paediatrics in a well informed manner. Whilst inactivity may still be the treatment of choice in certain cases, it should only be carried out with the full knowledge that all is well, and this obviously will involve the use and understanding of new investigations and techniques. In my opinion the authors have achieved their aims and though there are those who may always have reservations, they must surely accept the authors' appraisal of the modern approach to this science.

VICTOR R. TINDALL

Cardiff, 1971

PREFACE

This book confines itself to those aspects of pre-natal development which are of importance to the clinician. We hope to present a reasonably concise account of this relatively new and rapidly expanding field of medical science. Stress is given to concepts which may not yet be in many standard obstetric and paediatric texts. Also, we wish to provide an easily accessible collection of reference data for the busy member of junior staff to refer to during the course of his routine work. We therefore make no apology for any repetition needed to make each section readable without many cross references.

The selection of a title posed some difficulty and it is hoped that the one finally chosen proves acceptable. To some obstetricians such terms as ante-natal or pre-natal paediatrics suggest a growing proprietary interest on the part of the paediatrician in the pregnant woman.

References have, as far as possible, been excluded from the text and are inserted as an alphabetical list at the end of each chapter. Titles have been included to aid the teacher in his selection for further reading. In the case of the longer reference lists a few key references are set out under 'Guides to Further Reading'.

G. F. BATSTONE
A. W. BLAIR
J. M. SLATER

Bristol, 1971

ACKNOWLEDGEMENTS

We gratefully acknowledge the co-operation and advice of many people in the production of this book.

We wish to express our thanks to:

Our respective departments for tolerance and co-operation;

Mr. Victor R. Tindall, M.D., F.R.C.S., M.R.C.O.G., for critically reading the text and writing the foreword;

John W. Lockyer Esq., F.I.M.L.T., B.Sc., for help in the preparation of Chapter VI;

Miss Neeta M. Bampton, M.P.S., for help on the preparation of Chapter VII;

Miss Ann E. Fey, S.R.N., for help in the preparation of Chapter I;

Keith Longdon Esq., for photography and diagrams;

Miss Marina Warr and the secretarial staff of the Dept. of Child Health, Bristol, for patiently carrying out the secretarial work;

Mrs. Sheila Lambert for secretarial work;

The authors and publishers (separately acknowledged) who have granted permission for the reproduction of charts and diagrams;

The publishers of this book who have shown enormous co-operation, encouragement and patience.

CONTENTS

CHAPTER 1

A 'SKETCH-MAP' OF FETAL MORPHOLOGY AND FUNCTION

Intrauterine events during pregnancy move so fast and have so many facets that it is impossible to visualise all these at once. It therefore seemed appropriate to include a chapter at the beginning of this book to set out in very much simplified form some of the major events and landmarks in intrauterine development. As will be seen, this chapter in no sense competes with embryological texts and its main purpose is to create an impression of the overall process and to emphasise a few major points.

Embryologists divide intrauterine life into three main stages.

1. Pre-implantation processes.
2. Embryonic phase, from implantation until the processes of organogenesis are completed about the sixth week.
3. The fetal phase, which lasts until the pregnancy comes to an end.

These processes to some extent merge into one another, but they provide convenient milestones. Moreover, it is quite reasonable, for instance, to separate off the stage during which organogenesis takes place when considering the mechanism of production of congenital abnormality. Although it is convenient and simpler to consider separately the development of the various systems, it is to a large extent artificial, as they undergo their development simultaneously and interact with one another. For example the development of the adrenal cortex is hypoplastic in anencephalics, presumably because a pituitary is not developed.

EARLY DEVELOPMENT

The conceptus implants at the blastocyst stage about seven days after fertilization. It consists of a vacuolated clump of cells, of pin-head size, into which projects a clump of cells known as the inner cell mass. The inner cell mass differentiates into three layers, the ectoderm, the mesoderm, and the endoderm. The mesoderm grows outwards and lines the blastocyst. About this time two cavities appear within the inner cell mass, one in the ectoderm and the other in the endoderm forming, respectively, the amnion and the yolk sac. The inner cell mass then moves into the centre of the blastocyst cavity but remains attached to it by a stalk. The opposing layers of ectoderm and endoderm with the mesoderm interposed between them are destined to become the embryo.

Expansion of the amnion fills out the blastocyst obliterating the previous blastocyst cavity and engulfs the yolk sac. Thus ectoderm lines the amniotic cavity and forms an outer layer over the yolk sac and the stalk. What was previously the embryonic plate becomes rapidly more organised into symmetrical protuberances arranged along an axis which consists initially of a groove on the dorsal surface of the plate which later becomes the neural tube. By 25 days the conceptus is of such a shape that the forerunners of fetal structures can be recognized. To give the reader some idea about the size of the fetus (not the total intrauterine contents) at different intrauterine ages the Table 1.1 has been included. For more detailed consideration of intrauterine growth, see chapter 5.

PLACENTAL DEVELOPMENT AND STRUCTURE

The wall of the blastocyst cavity, known as the trophoblast, into which the inner cell mass projects, is formed of flattened cells,

TABLE 1.1 *Approximate size of fetus at different intrauterine ages.*

Age from conception, complete weeks	*Size cm*	*Stage*
0	Microscopic	Pre-implantation
2	0·02	Embryonic
3	0·15	
4	0·5	
5	0·8	
6	1·2	
8	3·0	Fetal
12	7·3	
16	15·7	
20	24	
24	30	
28	36	Potentially viable fetus

which during the process of implantation become differentiated into two layers. The outer layer is the syncytiotrophoblast and the inner layer the cytotrophoblast, or Langhan's layer. The trophoblast invades the endometrium and makes contact with maternal capillaries. The latter form the maternal placental circulation through the intervillous space. Into this space projections of the trophoblast grow. These are the villi, which are covered with syncytiotrophoblast and have a cytotrophoblastic core. These are seen at the beginning of the third week of development, but by the end of that week, the villi have a mesodermal core continuous with the mesoderm lining the blastocyst. Soon after this haemopoetic tissue and blood vessels appear in the villi, and together with similar differentiation in the body stalk and in the fetus itself, a continuous circulation is established.

When the mesodermal invasion of the trophoblast has occurred, the latter is named the chorion. This at first surrounds the whole blastocyst, but later develops further on the side adjacent to the uterine wall, whilst the remainder of the chorion atrophies. This localized chorion becomes the placenta. This is connected to the fetus by the umbilical cord which arises in the body stalk, and in this way vascular connections are established between the villi and the fetus.

As described earlier, the amnion expands to fill out the blastocyst. It takes with it its outer covering of mesoderm, and eventually fuses lightly with the peripheral chorion, where the villi have atrophied. This, of course, has its inner lining of mesoderm. The amnion and chorion form the membranes, and the spongy layer between them is thus mesodermal in origin.

This kind of placenta, where the villi are in direct contact with maternal blood with no endothelium present on the maternal side, is known as haemochorial, and is found in all anthropoids, and many other groups of mammals as well as in man.

The placenta is commonly attached to the posterior wall of the uterus near the fundus, depending on the site of implantation of the blastocyst. Occasionally a low attachment wholly or partly in the lower uterine segment may occur, described as placenta praevia. The mechanism which determines the site of implantation is not understood.

The umbilical cord, containing two arteries and one vein is usually inserted near the centre of the placenta but may be inserted at any point, including into the membranes (velamentous insertion).

For detailed anatomical description of the placenta, reference to a more comprehensive source is recommended. In brief, the maternal surface is divided into 15–30 cotyledons, and from it across the intervillous space containing maternal blood, pass anchoring villi, and irregularly distributed septae, to the outer wall of the space. The spiral arteries which supply maternal blood to the space appear to open at the base, or in the lower third of the septa. The fetal surface is covered with the single-layered amnion, beneath which are enclosed the larger branches of the umbilical vessels.

The spiral arteries lose their muscular coats in their terminal portions where they are lined only with endothelium.

AN OUTLINE OF PLACENTAL FUNCTION

The placenta and its membranes form a complex link between mother and fetus. It transports nutrient substances and oxygen to the fetus, and excretory products away from it, for elimination by the mother. The placenta also contains some kind of immunological barrier which allows separate development of the fetus. It may well be that defects in this barrier, which probably is in the maternal side of the placenta, will be shown to explain various abnormalities of pregnancy. The integrity of the placenta is essential to the growing fetus.

The placenta is also the site of intense biochemical activity, and the elaboration of hormones, enzymes, other complex proteins, carbohydrates, and lipid substances, has been demonstrated using histochemical techniques, and in vitro studies. Several of the hormones, e.g. oestrogens, progesterone, human chorionic gonadotrophin, and enzymes, e.g. alkaline phosphatase, can be measured in body fluids, and guide the clinician where he suspects abnormal placental function. The reader is referred to chapter 3, 'Assessment of Placental Function' for fuller details. It is interesting to note that oxygen consumption by the placenta per unit weight is twice that of the fetus. At term the placenta is around one-fifth the weight of the fetus but requires almost one-third of the oxygen consumed by the feto-placental unit.

Maternal blood spaces, eventually to become the intervillous space, become functional one to two weeks after implantation. At term the rate of flow through the intervillous space is 600–700 ml per minute.

In the syncytial cytotrophoblast covering the villi, lipoid inclusions are found which are probably related to the production of lipids, e.g. fatty acids and cholesterol, and to steroid synthesis. The presence of RNA is evidence of protein synthesis and many enzymes, e.g., phosphatases and respiratory enzymes, have been demonstrated. Also much glycogen is found; in contrast, the Langhan's layer is much less active, but is rich in iron.

The maternal side of the placenta, the basal plate, appears to be less concerned with fat and steroid production, but shows considerable evidence of protein synthesis, carbohydrates and enzymes.

The membranes, particularly the amnion, are metabolically

active. Transport of amniotic fluid occurs through the epithelium and intercellular spaces of the amnion. Systems of canaliculi and vacuoles have been demonstrated. The amnion may also be a site for steroid synthesis. Less is known about the activity of the chorion, but the spongy layer between the membranes can store large amounts of water. The relationship of this to amniotic fluid metabolism is not yet clear.

Despite the vast amount of investigation that has been directed to the human placenta, many theories on many different aspects remain conflicting, and a host of fascinating questions remain unanswered. The clinician must consider the fetus and placenta as a unit. He must also remember the maternal side of the placenta which is not shed in the third stage of labour. It is from here that the intervillous space receives its blood supply, maintenance of which is vital for the health of the fetus at all stages of pregnancy and labour. It also probably contains the immunological barrier, which prevents over-penetration of the trophoblast into maternal tissues, and, despite antigenic differences, allows the fetus to develop normally and separately.

UTERO-PLACENTAL PATHOLOGY

After the fetus is born, the delivered placenta is viewed and any macroscopic abnormalities noted. Some of these findings give useful information which may be correlated with the state of health of the fetus. Histological changes are mostly of interest as regards the aetiology of macroscopic changes.

Placental size. The placenta increases in size during pregnancy by continuous growth of the villi. In early pregnancy it is larger than the fetus and by about four months their weights are equal. After this time the fetus becomes increasingly larger until at term the placenta is about one-seventh of the fetal weight (range, one-fifth to one-tenth). Such figures vary with methods of weighing the placenta, viz. presence or absence of cord, membranes, and adherent blood clot. Placental weight correlates quite well with birthweight but there is better correlation between villous surface area and fetal size. In cases of hypertension and 'light-for-dates' infants the fetal weight, placental weight, and villous surface area are reduced. In Rhesus haemolytic disease the villous surface area has been found to be increased. When this condition is associated with hydrops fetalis the placenta is large, pale, friable, and oedematous. The degree of oedema and pallor are probably related to the extent of fetal anaemia. The placenta also tends to be large in diabetes and syphilis.

Degenerative changes. True placental infarction is now considered secondary to abnormalities of the maternal side of the placenta and adjoining uterus, as it is these structures which maintain the fetal placenta and fetus. The spiral arteries enter the centres of the fetal lobules and hence blood flows into the intervillous space to nourish the chorionic villi. In essential hypertension the basal and spiral arteries show a proliferative thickening of the vessel wall, thus narrowing the lumen and decreasing blood flow in the intervillous space. The changes in the spiral arteries are an exaggeration of the normal late pregnancy state but those of the basal arteries are specific for hypertension. In pre-eclampsia and eclampsia the arterial changes are similar to those of malignant hypertension leading to fibrinoid necrosis of the placental bed arteries.

When infarction of the delivered placenta has occurred it is usually lobular in distribution and associated with occlusion of more than one spiral artery. When associated with hypertension, haematoma of the placenta (usually found in the context of abruptio placentae) is possibly due to spasm of spiral arteries with vessel wall rupture. In other cases hormone imbalance, trauma, or folic acid deficiency have been cited as causes.

Focal fibrinoid deposition at sites of focal necrosis of villi, if extensive, may resemble chronic infarction. Similarly intervillous thrombosis, which is probably due to stasis of blood in aneurysmal spaces, when old and widespread may resemble an old infarct. This lesion is so common as to be considered normal.

Of these lesions only true infarction and haematoma are of clinical importance as they are associated with fetal mortality.

The reduced villous surface area of the placenta in hypertension is seen as due to reduced blood flow caused by changes in the placental bed arteries. In hypertension the volume of the fetal capillary bed is high whereas in 'light-for-dates' infants both the fetal capillary volume and villous surface area are low. Hypoplasia of the vessels supplying the placenta has been proposed as the cause of the findings in the latter.

Septal cysts, when present, have been shown to be a sign of maturity in uncomplicated singleton pregnancies.

Radiologically calcification can be seen well before 35 weeks, increasing with length of gestation and tending to diminish on postmaturity. Histologically however calcification is difficult to demonstrate before 35 weeks and is progressive until term. There is little correlation between histological calcification and pre-eclampsia.

Histological examination of the placenta is not very reliable because there is variation in findings in different regions of the placenta and in relation to intervillous circulation. Caution is therefore required in assessing the significance of syncitial knots (which may be confused with syncitial sprouts), villus basement membrane thickening, fibrinoid necrosis, fetal vessel endarteritis and stromal fibrosis, some of which have been associated with hypertension.

However, proliferation of Langhan's cells, which are dependent on maternal blood supply, and their differentiation into large cytotrophoblasts is a good index of chronic placental ischaemia.

Infection. When bacteria ascend from the vagina as may occur after rupture of the membranes, they may infect the placenta, which then responds by forming a polymorph exudate. Such placentitis is rare.

In tuberculosis when the fetus is infected, some evidence may be found of tuberculous lesions on the placenta and membranes.

The syphilitic placenta may appear normal but that of the

stillborn syphilitic fetus is bulky, pale and fibrotic. These large placentas show a proliferative fibrosis and sometimes spirochaetes may be demonstrated.

Umbilical cord. The presence in the umbilical cord of only one umbilical artery is frequently associated with chromosomal or other abnormalities. This finding seems less significant in twins.

DEVELOPMENT OF MAIN SYSTEMS

The cardiovascular system. Is derived from mesoderm by its differentiation into angioblastic tissue which forms blood vessels and corpuscles during the third week from conception. The vascular pattern is at first symmetrical, the precursor of the heart being formed by the fusion of paired vessels which then fold in a complex manner to form a structure with chambers by the end of the sixth week. By this time it is already beating and pumping blood, although the valvular mechanism and conducting systems are not developed at this stage. The latter appears initially as the atrio-ventricular node at the end of the fifth week.

The blood. The development of cellular elements and the changes in their sites of production are summarized in Fig. 1.1.

The iron required for haemoglobin synthesis is actively taken up from the mother. The level of plasma iron in the fetus at birth is greater than that in the mother and this reflects the iron storing process necessary for post-natal haemoglobin synthesis. The earliest haemoglobin is known as embryonic haemoglobin about which relatively little is known. The main haemoglobin throughout pregnancy is fetal haemoglobin (HbF) and this accounts for some 95 per cent of the total. HbF is better suited to the fetal oxygen tension than adult haemoglobin. This latter starts to be produced in the last few weeks of pregnancy and its level increases rapidly after term.

Many of the blood group antigens, e.g. the rhesus groups, are found early in fetal life but others, e.g. group A, may not be much in evidence even at birth.

FIG. 1.1. *The development of the cellular elements of the blood and their sites of production (from Clinical Haematology. Wintrobe, M. M. 1967).*

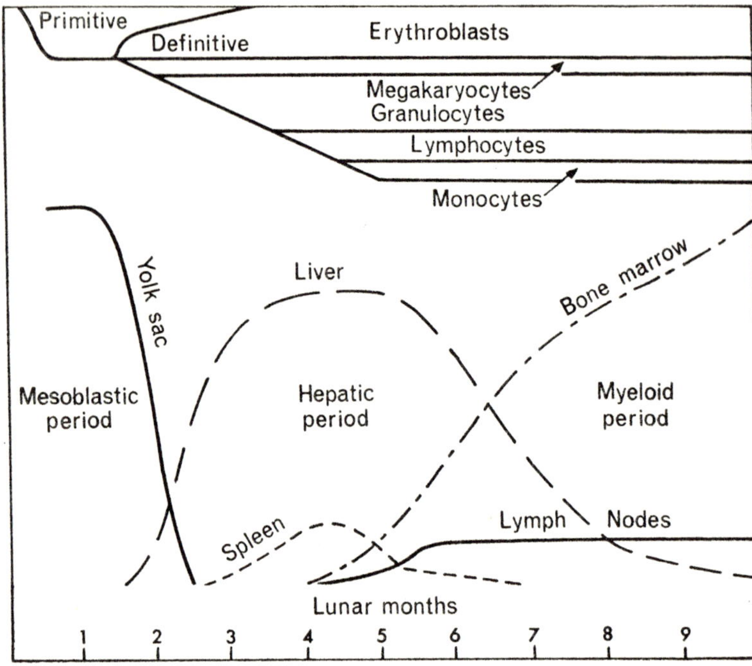

Immunological system. The thymus gland contains lymphoid tissue from about 12 weeks, and the spleen and lymph nodes soon after 20 weeks. Proper germinal centres do not normally develop until after birth.

IgM is detectable in the fetus at about 12 weeks and may increase in response to infection. IgG in the fetus is almost all of maternal origin although there is evidence that by about 6 months the fetus is capable of synthesising IgG. Of the maternal antibodies, only those which are IgG are transported across the placenta and these are present in the fetal circulation at concentrations which are the same, or slightly higher, than in the maternal circulation. These maternal antibodies provide immunity to many infections, particularly virus infections, e.g. rubella.

The respiratory system. The lungs are formed by budding from the foregut and their endothelial elements are therefore formed from endoderm. These lung buds are formed by the thirty-second day when the embryo is 5 mm long. A bronchial tree and air passages are formed by subsidiary budding by the sixth week but the potential air spaces are not formed until 24 weeks of gestation. In early pregnancy the lining epithelium is cuboidal and ciliated epithelium appears about 18 weeks. This becomes flattened into squamous epithelium by 28 weeks, by which time the pulmonary capillaries have become more closely applied to the alveoli. At this stage gaseous exchange becomes a possibility.

The presumptive air spaces are fluid-filled and this fluid is taken in from the liquor amnii and is absorbed through the pulmonary epithelium. Respiratory movements have been observed at 12 weeks and these may assist in this process, although the quantities of fluid involved are probably quite small.

Relatively late in pregnancy, about 36 weeks, a lipoid substance termed surfactant can be detected in the fetal lungs. The surface tension lowering properties of this substance play an important role in preventing alveolar collapse at full expiration after birth.

Central nervous system. Development of the nervous system begins with the appearance of the neural plate at the third week of intrauterine life. As this plate folds into a tube, distinct groups of cells form along each edge to form paired structures called the neural crests. These then migrate to a dorso-lateral position and form the cells of the spinal sensory ganglia. These cells then develop two processes, one centrally-growing which penetrates into the neural tube itself and another growing peripherally. The latter, together with processes growing outwards from the anterior horn cells, forms the peripheral nerve.

Myelinisation in the peripheral nerves is accomplished by the neurilemmal cells and commences about the fourth month of intrauterine life. These neurilemmal, or Schwann cells originate in the spinal sensory ganglia and spread peripherally to enwrap bundles of axons numbering from one to twenty.

Myelinisation within the cord is a different process and is accomplished by oligodendroglial cells. This also begins about the fourth intrauterine month but some of the tracts are not fully myelinated until the first or second post-natal years.

The autonomic nervous system derives from cells termed sympathochromaffin tissue which originates from the neural crests. The smaller cells in this tissue differentiate further into sympathetic nerve cells and the larger ones into the chromaffin cells.

Endocrine system. The pituitary is formed by ectoderm from two different sources. The anterior pituitary is formed from the ectoderm of Rathke's pouch in the roof of the mouth and the posterior pituitary arises from neuroectoderm. A.C.T.H. has been demonstrated as early as the tenth week in the pituitary.

The thyroid gland makes its appearance in the latter half of the fourth week as an outgrowth from a diverticulum which extends ventrally from the pharynx (an area corresponding to the back of the tongue). It migrates caudally, and receives contributions from the fourth pharyngeal pouches. By the nineteenth week it is functional.

The fetal adrenal cortex appears from the root of the mesentery early in the sixth week. Its development is probably dependent on the proper development of the pituitary. The cortex is rather different from the adult one in that it contains a fetal zone which disappears rapidly post-natally and the steroid hormones produced are more numerous than in the adult. The precise sequence of its functions is complex and fascinating and the fetal pituitary-adrenal axis may have a crucial role in determining the length of pregnancy.

Cortisol levels in the fetus are lower than in maternal circulation despite the fact that cortisol crosses the placenta. This is due to low levels of cortisol carriage proteins and to the rapid metabolism of cortisol in the fetus.

Locomotor system. The limb buds are discernible at 37 days of gestation and the structures destined to form the hip joint at 5–6 weeks. There is evidence of muscular activity at about 10 weeks and this may be the mechanism whereby the cavities of the joints are produced.

The gut. The 'folding off' of the embryonic plate encloses part of the endodermal cavity, the yolk sac, within what is then the embryo. This endoderm is destined to become the gut, extending from the oral membrane at the cephalic end to the cloacal membrane caudally. Parenchyma of liver, lung, and pancreas are formed by outgrowths from it. The stomach first appears about the fifth week as a midline dilatation in the tube. It differentiates lesser and greater curvatures and at the same time the gut increases in length. The increase in body cavity contents forces some of this developing gut out into the umbilical cord, a process which is permitted by, or stimulates the formation of a long dorsal mesentery. Rotation of the gut starts at this stage and is complete when the gut returns to the peritoneal cavity during the third month. Before 'folding off' occurs a diverticulum appears from the yolk sac which forms, after folding off, a diverticulum stretching from the hindgut into the umbilical cord. This, termed the allantois, joins at its caudal end the hindgut, to form a dilatation termed the cloaca (see paragraph on Genito-urinary system). Part of the cloacal membrane goes on to form the anus and this is patent about the eighth week of intrauterine life.

Maltase, sucrase, and isomaltase are detectable in gut mucosa by about three months and achieve normal levels at about seven months. Lactase is present in full concentrations about term.

Genito-urinary system. By the end of the third week the primitive gut is attached to the posterior wall of the body cavity by a mesentery. On either side of this is the intermediate cell mass of mesoderm, the medial part of which proliferates to form the urogenital ridge. From this are derived the whole of the genital and urinary systems except the vulva, bladder, and urethra.

These latter structures originate in the cloaca, the lower end of the primitive gut.

The urogenital ridges appear about the fourth and fifth weeks and in them differentiated gonads, ovaries, or testes, can be seen by the sixth week. The germinal layers of oogonia, or spermatogonia are believed to originate from the yolk sac as early as the first three weeks of life and migrate through the mesentery to reach the gonads.

Lateral to the gonads, at the beginning of the fourth week, the first of a series of tubules is formed at the upper end of the urogenital ridges. These tubules, known as the pronephros, disappear by the end of the fifth week, but their duct, the Wolffian duct, which passes down through the ridge to the cloaca, persists to drain a second set of tubules, the mesonephros, which develop lower down the ridge. These appear during the fifth week and have degenerated by the seventh week. They partly persist in the male as the vasa efferentia and the rete testis, and in the female, occasionally, as functionless vestiges in the broad ligament.

Near the end of the fifth week a third system of tubules develops even further down the ridge in its caudal part. This is the metanephros, and from this the renal cortex and medulla develop. From the persisting pronephric (Wolffian) duct, a diverticulum grows up from near where the duct opens into the cloaca. This contributes to the calyces, renal pelvis, and ureter, and fuses with the cap of metanephric mesoderm to form the fetal kidney. This process occurs on each side. The kidney is at first caudal, but later (probably due to increased growth of the lower end of the fetus) appears to grow headwards.

The ureter eventually opens into the cloaca, separately from the Wolffian duct. The latter, in the male, persists as the vas deferens and the epididymis whereas in the female it largely degenerates to appear vestigially as Gärtner's duct, in the broad ligament and vaginal wall.

The paramesonephric (Müllerian) duct from which most of the female reproductive system is derived, develops at the beginning of the sixth week in the intermediate cell mass, lateral to the Wolffian duct. The Müllerian duct on each side, grows down caudally, and bends medially to come into opposition with its partner, and later, at the end of the second month to fuse with it. The upper non-fused parts form the two fallopian tubes, and the lower portions, now a single cavity, become the uterus. Downgrowths, called vaginal bulbs, are produced which are at first solid, but later canalised, form the upper part of the vagina.

In the male the Müllerian ducts atrophy, but the lower fused parts persist as the prostatic utricle, the male uterus, which opens into the prostatic urethra.

The endodermal cloaca is divided by the urorectal septum, into hindgut and urogenital sinus. The latter forms the lower vagina, the urethra and the urinary bladder. The prostate gland is formed in the third month from urethral outgrowths. In the female these are represented as the rudimentary para-urethral glands.

The external genitalia are also derived from the cloaca.

RENAL FUNCTION AND BODY FLUIDS

The total body water as a percentage of total body weight is higher in infants than adults. The extracellular fluid volume is large especially in premature infants, when it may represent more than 40 per cent of the body weight.

Urine is formed by the fetus from the fourth month of gestation and voided into the amniotic fluid. Although the fetal kidney shows morphological maturity by about 36 weeks full physiological maturity is not attained until 1 year of age. The urine formed in utero is very dilute and at birth is hypotonic to the plasma. The newborn infant (especially if premature) is less able than the adult to conserve water or excrete a water load. The glomerular filtration rate is low and, as the renal plasma flow is lower, the filtration fraction is very high. The neonate has great difficulty in excreting a salt load and this calls for great care during parenteral fluid therapy.

The acid-base balance of the fetus in the presence of good placental function is ultimately regulated by the maternal lungs and kidneys. The newborn has a less dependable hyperpnoea in acidosis and in addition the ability of the kidney to excrete hydrogen ion is limited.

The renal threshold for bicarbonate is lower in the newborn than in the adult and this probably accounts for the low bicarbonate and high chloride levels in the serum of infants. The low phosphate excretion at birth is a continuation of the phosphate conservation in utero when the serum phosphate level is higher than that of the mother.

Despite these limitations of the kidney at birth it has adequate function except in abnormal situations.

BROWN ADIPOSE TISSUE

Brown adipose tissue differs from normal white adipose tissue by having many mitochondria and multiple small fat globules in the cell. It is found mostly in the neck, axillae, groins, and around many thoracic and abdominal organs. Brown adipose tissue is detectable in the human fetus from 28 weeks and increases in amount until term. The function of this tissue is to provide heat by metabolism of the fat globules thus dispensing with the need for shivering. Control of metabolism seems to be via the sympathetic nervous system and heat is produced locally by metabolism of the fat by the mitochondria without the fatty acids being released into the circulation. Brown adipose tissue provides a heat source for the newborn infant without utilizing glycogen stores for purely thermogenic purposes.

ENERGY SUPPLY IN THE FETUS

Maternal glucose freely passes across the placenta and is the principal substrate for energy metabolism. Fatty acids and ketone bodies pass less readily across the placenta. It is believed that the fetus can to some extent metabolize ketone bodies but not fatty acids. Glucose is also used to form glycogen stores in the fetus and by about 20 weeks the liver contains adult concentrations of glycogen and the concentration increases greatly towards term. In addition both skeletal muscle and cardiac muscle contain large glycogen stores at birth. These glycogen stores are an important energy source after birth as at this time fatty acids are metabolized very little and the enzymes of gluconeogenesis are present at only low levels. These glycogen stores are easily mobilized, and may be utilized within 24 hours of birth. Glycogen reserves may also be used before birth if the fetal oxygen supply is impaired and anaerobic glycolysis is required. If the cause of impaired oxygen supply is placental malfunction then the glucose supply is also decreased and hence glycogen stores are used. This explains why glycogen reserves are low in some 'light-for-dates' infants and after certain obstetric complications. It should be remembered that glycogen reserves are much lower in premature than full term infants. Lipogenesis from pyruvate and acetate in fetal liver is much more active than in the adult. Fetal subcutaneous lipid stores show much increase in the last few weeks of gestation. This subcutaneous fat acts both as a supply of metabolic energy and as insulation. Although the enzymes of lipolysis have been demonstrated in the fetus they are not usually activated until some hours after birth. This activation may be associated with the changes in hormone secretion.

BIOCHEMICAL DEVELOPMENT OF THE LIVER AT TERM

The degree of specialization of organs and the environment of the fetus change as pregnancy proceeds and in parallel with this many enzymes are induced or repressed. Alteration of hepatic enzyme activities near term equip the fetus for extrauterine life. These are of importance to the clinician as such enzymes may be present in insufficient amounts in the prematurely delivered or the unhealthy fetus.

Carbohydrate metabolism. There is evidence of glycogen synthesis by about 12 weeks of gestation and the hepatic glycogen concentration increases to give high levels at term. The enzymes of glycogen degradation to glucose show little activity during most of fetal life but can be activated if required. This usually occurs at term and in response to hypoxia. There is evidence to suggest that the fetal pituitary and adrenal cortex play an important role in development of some enzymes of glycogen metabolism. The aerobic glycolysis rate is similar in the fetus and adult but the fetus is able to produce more lactate during anaerobic glycolysis than the adult.

Evidence from animal studies indicates that the key enzymes of gluconeogenesis (the method by which the liver converts amino acids and pyruvate to glucose during starvation) although present in the fetus have little activity until after birth. They may be activated by glucagon or adrenaline. Some studies suggest that the ability of the liver to metabolize galactose is very great at term.

Nitrogen metabolism. Synthesis of albumin in fetal liver has been demonstrated at 3–4 months. However, the levels of albumin, lipoproteins, and the hepatic coagulation factors tend to be low at birth, particularly in premature infants. The ability to break down certain amino acids such as phenylalanine and tyrosine is rather low in infants at term and more so in premature infants.

Detoxication mechanisms. The enzymes of glucuronide conjugation and excretion develop towards the end of gestation but at term are still well below adult levels. These enzymes are required for excretion of bile, chloramphenicol, morphine, adrenal steroids etc. Similarly, other detoxication systems of the liver such as oxidative, acetylation, and sulphation detoxication show low activity at birth. Administration of phenobarbitone has been shown to increase the levels of conjugation enzymes in the infant liver when given to mother or neonate (see also chapter 7).

POINTS USEFUL TO THE PATHOLOGIST IN ASSESSING FETAL AGE

The general appearance of the fetus, its length and weight are useful guides to age. In addition the nature of the skin is often of help. At about 28 weeks of gestation the skin is red and wrinkled, lanugo is present and there is very little subcutaneous fat. By 36 weeks the red colour of the skin has largely faded and the nails reach the ends of the digits. At term the lanugo has disappeared, the skin feels thicker because of the presence of subcutaneous fat and the nails project beyond the finger tips. These superficial features are a poor guide with 'light-for-dates' babies. In these infants the brain is large relative to the size of the liver.

Some histological features are more constant.

Lung. Until 20 weeks of gestation the bronchi and bronchioles are lined by columnar and the alveolae by cuboidal epithelium. At this stage few vessels are found adjacent to the alveolar epithelium. At about 28 weeks the alveolar epithelium is flattened and vessels are found adjacent to it.

Kidney. The kidneys of immature fetuses show a nephrogenic zone, comprising immature glomeruli, in the cortex. These immature glomeruli are not found when the baby weighs more than about 2,500 g, which is usually at 34–36 weeks of gestation.

Liver. In the immature fetus the hepatic arteries, portal veins and bile ducts are surrounded by relatively large amounts of mesenchymal tissue and there are many prominent foci of erythropoiesis. At term there are a few small islands of erythropoietic tissue remaining and the liver cells pack more closely to the hepatic vessels. In a normal fetus glycogen may be found from about 20 weeks and increases in quantity until term. This is an unreliable guide to maturity as much glycogen may be utilized during delivery and glycogen levels are low in 'light-for-dates' babies.

References and guides to further reading

Aherne, W., and Dunnill, M. S. (1966). 'Quantitative aspects of placental structure', *J. Path. Bact.*, **91**, 123.

Auricchio, S., Rubino, A., and Murset, G. (1965). 'Intestinal glycosidase activities in the human embryo, fetus and newborn', *Pediatrics*, **35**, 944.

BERG, T., and NILSSON, B. A. (1969). 'Fetal development of serum levels of IgG and IgM', *Acta Pediat. Scand.*, **58**, 577.

BILLINGTON, W. D. (1967). 'Transplantation immunity and the placenta', *J. Obstet. Gynaec. Br. Commw.*, **74**, 834.

BROSENS, I., ROBERTSON, W. B., and DIXON, H. G. (1967). 'The physiological response of the vessels of the placental bed to normal pregnancy', *J. Path. Bact.*, **93**, 569.

BROWN, N. J. (1960). 'Pathology of the premature infant', *Prematurity*, Corner, B. (London: Cassell).

DAWKINS, M. J. R. (1966). 'Developing function in newborn mammalian liver', *Br. Med. Bull.*, **22**, 27.

HSIA, D. Y. (1968). *Human Developmental Genetics* (Chicago: Year Book Medical Publishers).

HULL, D. (1966). 'Structure and function of brown adipose tissue', *Br. Med. Bull.*, **22**, 92.

JOST, A., and PICON, L. (1970). 'Hormonal control of fetal development and metabolism', *Adv. Metab. Dis.*, **4**, 123.

MACNAUGHTON, M. C. (1969). 'Endocrinology of the foetus', *Foetus and Placenta*, eds. Klopper, A., and Diczfalusy, E. (Oxford: Blackwell Scientific Publications).

MILLER, J. F. A. P. (1966). 'Immunity in the foetus and newborn', *Br. Med. Bull.*, **22**, 21.

POTTER, E. C. (1961). *Pathology of the Fetus and the Infant* (Chicago: Year Book Medical Publishers).

ROBERTSON, W. B., and DIXON, H. G. (1969). 'Uteroplacental pathology', *The Fetus and Placenta*, eds. Klopper, A., and Diczfalusy, E. (Oxford: Blackwell Scientific Publications).

SHELLEY, H. J. (1969). 'The energy supply of the fetus in normal and abnormal circumstances', *Perinatal Medicine*, eds. Huntingford, P. J., Huter, E. A., and Saling, E. (Stuttgart: Georg Thieme Verlag).

THOMSEN, K., and HIERSCHE, H-D. (1969). 'The functional morphology of the placenta, the foetus, the membranes and the umbilical cord', *Foetus and Placenta*, eds. Klopper, A., and Diczfalusy, E. (Oxford: Blackwell Scientific Publications).

WIGGLESWORTH, J. S. (1969). 'Vascular anatomy of the human placenta and its significance for placental pathology', *J. Obstet. Gynaec. Br. Commonw.*, **76**, 979.

WINTROBE, M. M. (1967). *Clinical Haematology* (London: Henry Kimpton).

CHAPTER 2

ADAPTATION TO THE NEWBORN STATE: FETAL MONITORING

Although the identifiable hazards of extrauterine existence seem to be more than those facing the fetus, it is not correct to regard the fetus as totally protected or of having its physiological functions performed for it. It is a complex organism which is well adapted to its particular environment. This environment changes enormously throughout gestation and the products of conception are vastly different by the time term is reached. An outline of some of these changes is given in the previous chapter.

Probably the most significant change in this environment is the event of birth, requiring as it does a rapid transition to a free living state without the luxury of a placenta as an organ of respiration and excretion and in which the newborn child must govern its own homeostasis. The circulation must radically alter its dynamics and 'dormant' organ systems must become active in a relatively short space of time. It is true that the first breath is taken within seconds or minutes of delivery and the haemodynamics change over abruptly, but the complete processes take considerably longer, even in the cardiovascular and respiratory systems.

When delivery takes place the circulation is rearranged from a system of pumps in parallel to a system of pumps in series by three principal events which are initiated at birth, namely, the closure of the foramen ovale, the closure of the ductus arteriosus and the obliteration of the placental circulation.

The first breath sharply raises the oxygen tension in the blood and this has been shown experimentally to produce vasodilation of the pulmonary vascular bed which will in turn lower the pulmonary vascular resistance and thus the right-sided pressure. This must presumably be sufficient to overcompensate the increased flow through the lungs due to the occlusion of the placental circulation. If the cord is clamped late the fetus receives a larger volume of placental transfusion in the approximate (but very variable) order of 80–100 ml; and pulmonary pressures are higher.

The increase in the oxygen tension may also act as a trigger mechanism for closure of the ductus arteriosus which constricts, thus allowing the now increasing divergence of pressures between the right and left sides of the circulation.

Occlusion of the cord removes the left-to-right shunt of the placenta thus raising the left-sided pressure and causing the foramen ovale flap valve to close.

Several conditions are necessary for the taking of the first breath:

1. Integrity of the central nervous arrangements responsible for the cyclical activity of respiration.
2. Integrity of peripheral chemoreceptors.
3. Histologically mature lung containing surfactant.
4. A clear or clearable airway.
5. The peripheral stimuli of being born.

The fluid in the lung at birth probably facilitates the first breath although its resistive properties are greater than those in the inflated lung.

The numerous mechanisms of preservation of the internal milieu effect the change to extra uterine existence in different ways. The kidneys, as already mentioned, excrete urine throughout a large part of fetal life and are able to cope with the usual processes after birth, but do not possess the full capacity of the adult kidney for a year or so after birth, having a lower blood flow and poorer solute concentrating power.

Temperature, on the other hand, changes abruptly at birth which calls hitherto unused processes into action, such as shivering and the metabolism of brown adipose tissue. The vascular system also has a vital role to play as vasoconstriction can conserve heat and if this is impaired (as may happen with gross cerebral insult) heat may be lost very rapidly.

The main source of energy is from carbohydrate of which the fetus has relatively small stores. Premature and 'light-for-dates' infants have less in the way of stores and are at greater risk from hypoglycaemia, although the risk for the two groups is different as prematures have lower and 'light-for-dates' higher metabolic rates than the term infant.

During anoxia, due to placental insufficiency or separation energy is supplied from glycogen by anaerobic metabolism. This is less efficient than aerobic metabolism by a factor of eight (if the criterion used is the amount of adenosine triphosphate made available). Anaerobic resources are not limitless and this form of metabolism produces a metabolic deficit which must be paid off later by respiration and aerobic metabolism. Nonetheless it is of great value to the fetus during parturition to be able to live on metabolic credit when the airways are not yet functioning and the integrity of the placenta is threatened or disrupted.

Anaerobic metabolism takes place in a situation of low oxygen tension when the non-availability of gaseous exchange causes the carbon dioxide tension to rise and it produces acid by-products which cause a lowering of bicarbonate and produce an acid pH in the blood. When the child is born and respiration is established, normal metabolism using oxygen and taking place via the tricarboxylate acid cycle (Krebs) renders anaerobic processes unnecessary, the excess CO_2 is eliminated via the lungs and normal levels of pO_2, pCO_2, bicarbonate, and pH are achieved. The kidneys of the fetus and newborn are less able than the adult kidney to help in an acidotic situation as their capacity to secrete hydrogen ion is less.

It is often of use clinically to know the extent of the metabolic deficit incurred by an infant during the course of labour as an index of how much leeway may be allowed before intervention by the obstetrician.

Some aspects of fetal metabolism seem to be specifically suited to the process of delivery. The fetus is better able than the adult to perform anaerobic respiration which is affected by metabolism of carbohydrate to lactate.

FETAL BLOOD SAMPLING

As stated earlier, the large stores of tissue glycogen at term allow the fetus to withstand relatively long periods of hypoxia. However, if the oxygen supply is insufficient to allow the final stages of glucose utilization to occur, lactic acid accumulates. The pH is lowered, glycolysis is inhibited, and less energy is available.

The detection of fetal acidosis has been used for the intrapartum assessment of fetal well-being. A pH below 7·20 is considered abnormal and suggestive of fetal hypoxia. During labour the fetal pH is fairly constant until it declines just before delivery to values between 7·35 and 7·25.

Techniques have been developed to measure fetal pH and thus, when performed at intervals during labour, have become a useful aid in assessing the significance of 'classical' fetal distress, viz. abnormal fetal heart rates and/or meconium in the liquor. Indications for the use of these methods include situations where fetal distress has already occurred and in 'at risk' pregnancies, where fetal distress or hypoxia is likely, e.g. pre-eclampsia, prolonged pregnancy, 'light-for-dates' babies.

The measurement is made on capillary blood from the fetal scalp. The membranes must be ruptured, and an endoscope is passed through the cervix and rested against the fetal scalp. By means of a guarded blade, manufactured for the purpose, a drop of blood is allowed to collect and is then removed using a heparinized glass capillary tube. Analysis of the sample is performed using an Astrup machine. This apparatus can, if necessary, measure the pCO_2, pO_2 and base excess, using Siggaard-Andersen nomogram charts. The pH values provide the most useful criteria of fetal acidosis. Occasionally it may be necessary to measure the base excess, to distinguish between an acidosis originating in the mother (known as an infusion acidosis) from a true primary hypoxic fetal acidosis. If there is a negative base excess (base deficit) of less than 3·0 mEq/l, it is probable that the acidosis is maternal in origin. Incoordinate uterine action, dehydration, and ketosis, can cause maternal acidosis.

Other problems have been encountered using the method, particularly concerning the collection of the fetal blood sample. Contamination of the sample with liquor, and prolonged exposure of it to air, lower and raise the pH respectively. Congestion of the scalp due to a caput or pressure of the endoscope may also affect results. It has been questioned whether scalp blood is representative of the circulation in general.

Much has been published during the six years of its use in the U.K., mainly by a small group of workers, yet few centres are using it routinely. Impressive figures showing the reduction in numbers of caesarean sections for fetal distress have been produced, but the correlation between pH and Apgar scores at birth is much less convincing. There is no doubt that our understanding of feto-maternal physiology has been increased by these studies, but it remains to be seen whether perinatal mortality and morbidity are reduced in large obstetric populations over long periods.

FETAL HEART MONITORING

Auscultation of the fetal heart has been the time-honoured way of confirming fetal life both before and during labour. However, in both situations, this examination is infrequent and carried out for extremely short periods of time. Considerable evaluation of the techniques of *continuous* fetal heart monitoring, particularly during labour, is now being undertaken. The standard criteria of fetal distress as shown by fetal heart rate alterations, e.g. greater than 160 beats per minute, less than 120 beats per minute etc. are being replaced by more complex definitions and interpretations.

Methods. The following methods have been used.

1. Phonocardiography.
2. Indirect and direct fetal electrocardiography.
3. Ultrasonic Doppler effect.

Whichever method is used, it is usual to relate the recorded heart rates to uterine contractions, and the latter are recorded by external tocograph or intrauterine sensor. The tocograph is a device which can be fixed to the maternal abdomen, and can be incorporated in the same apparatus as the heart rate monitor.

Phonocardiography uses a microphone attached to the maternal abdomen. Apparatus has been manufactured which records the heart rate changes as tracings, and incorporates filters to exclude unwanted sounds.

Indirect fetal electrocardiography involves the use of electrodes placed over the maternal abdomen. Composite fetal and maternal complexes are obtained, which reduce the usefulness of the technique. Direct fetal electrocardiography, where an electrode is directly applied to the presenting part of the fetus is now more commonly used. Various appliances have been developed using clips, suction, or 'Araldite' glue, for fixing electrodes to the fetal scalp. Recorded fetal heart rates and irregularities can be monitored, and computers have been used for the more complex analysis and interpretation of these patterns.

Similar continuous recordings can be obtained using ultrasonic detectors utilizing the Doppler effect. These are extremely useful for the early detection of fetal life, but because of the directional quality of the sound waves produced, are more difficult to use continuously. Doubts have been expressed concerning their prolonged use, as chromosome breakages have been shown to occur in in vitro studies on human cells (see also chapter 7).

Heart rate patterns

1. *Baseline fetal heart rate.* The normal range is between 120 and 160 beats per minute, and is measured between contractions. Rapid persistent irregularities from beat to beat, up to 25 beats per minute, have been considered as part of the normal pattern, but these can hardly be detected by ordinary auscultation.

2. *Periodic (or transient) changes.* These are accelerations or decelerations lasting longer than 20 seconds during which the rate is outside the 120–160 beats per minute range, or varies more than 30 beats per minute from the baseline fetal heart rate. Tachycardia is thus described in the accelerations, and bradycardia in the decelerations.

3. *Prolonged variations.* Those lasting more than 10 minutes. Slowing of the heart rate and its relationship to uterine contractions is important.

4. *Early deceleration.* (Type 1, or head compression dip): occurs at the beginning of a contraction.

5. *Delayed (late) deceleration.* (Type 2, or utero-placental insufficiency dip): occurs not less than 30 seconds *after* the onset of a contraction.

6. *Variable deceleration.* (Type 0, or cord compression dip, some workers call this type 3): occurs with no fixed time-relationship to contractions.

The interpretation of these patterns is the subject of much controversy and discussion, as is their application to everyday obstetric problems. Delayed decelerations, and prolonged variations, either persistent tachycardia or bradycardia, suggest fetal hypoxia.

It is clear that these sophisticated methods of fetal heart monitoring cannot be used in isolation, and the observations made should be interpreted in conjunction with the whole range of clinical and biochemical information that is available to the clinician.

References and guides to further reading

ASTRUP, P., JORGENSEN, K., SIGGARD-ANDERSEN, O., and ENGELL, K. (1960). 'The acid-base metabolism: a new approach', *Lancet*, **1**, 1035.

DAWES, G. S. (1968). 'Foetal and neonatal physiology' (Chicago: Medical Year Book Publishers).

GARUD, M. A., MAY, D. P. L., and SIMMONS, S. C. (1969). 'Foetal blood sampling in the regional hospital', *Br. Med. J.*, **1**, 346.

HUNTINGFORD, P., and PENDLETON, H. J. (1969). 'The clinical application of cardiotocography', *J. Obstet. Gynaec. Br. Commonw.*, **76**, 586.

LIND, J., STERN, L., and WEGELIUS, C. E. (1964). 'Human foetal and neonatal circulation' (Springfield Ill.: C. C. Thomas).

MORRIS, E. D., and BEARD, R. W. (1965). 'The rationale and technique of foetal blood sampling and amnioscopy', *J. Obstet. Gynaec. Br. Commonw.*, **72**, 489.

PENDLETON, H. J. (1970). 'Fetal heart monitoring', *Br. J. Hospt. Med.*, **3**, 509.

SALING, E., and SCHNEIDER, D. (1967). 'Biochemical supervision of the fetus during labour', *J. Obstet. Gynaec. Br. Commonw.*, **74**, 799.

TINDALL, V. R. (1970). 'The diagnosis and management of anoxia of the foetus', *Update*, **2**, 403.

WALSH, S. Z., and LIND, J. (1970). 'Physiology of the perinatal period', p. 141, ed. Stave, U. (New York: Appleton Century Crofts).

CHAPTER 3

ASSESSMENT OF PLACENTAL FUNCTION

Introduction

Much of this chapter deals with complex laboratory techniques. It should be emphasized that until resources and improvements in technique are such that all pregnant women can be screened, their use is limited by careful appraisal of the clinical situation.

All these methods have the common goal of reducing perinatal mortality, and the diagnosis of the fetus 'at risk' is all important. In this chapter, the emphasis is on the fetus during the ante-natal period, but obviously this will affect the condition during labour and the first weeks of life.

TABLE 3.1. *Fetal deaths (as a percentage).*

		Total
Stillbirths		
Before labour	27	
First stage	23	64
Second stage	14	
First week deaths		
First day	20	36
Second-seventh day	16	

As can be seen from the Table 3.1 more than a quarter of fetal deaths occur before labour has started.

The first step is the recognition of the 'at risk' fetus as early as possible in pregnancy, and then the initiation of ante-natal care and arrangements for delivery in a major unit under consultant care. Table 3.2 summarizes the risks, some of which (e.g. the light-for-dates baby and multiple pregnancy), will become apparent as pregnancy progresses.

TABLE 3.2. *A summary of risks.*

Mother	*Fetus*
Primigravida	Prematurity
Gravida 4 +	Light-for-dates
Increasing age	Multiple pregnancy
Poor obstetric history	Malpresentations
Low social class	Premature rupture of membranes
Poor clinic attender	Prolonged pregnancy
Hypertension (pre-eclampsia, essential hypertension)	
Renal disease	
Diabetes	
Severe cardiac disease	
Blood group incompatibilities	
Anaemia	
Haemoglobinopathies	
Threatened abortion	
Antepartum haemorrhage	

Table 3.3 shows the great disadvantages of an abnormal, 'poor', obstetric history.

TABLE 3.3 *Perinatal mortality according to previous obstetric history (after Butler and Bonham) (100 = average mortality).*

Obstetric history	*Parity* 0	1	2	3	4
Abortions or ectopics	127	116	150	155	173
Premature live births		153	148	157	186
Stillbirths/neonatal deaths		202	192	222	245
'Toxaemia'		96	130	135	184
Antepartum haemorrhage		133	199	140	143
Caesarean section		162	180	367	263

Knowledge gained from investigation of placental function gives the clinician valuable information which may help him reduce the risks associated with some causes of perinatal mortality. Needless to say it must be placed in the context of efficient and comprehensive ante-natal care. The subject is dealt with in two sections discussing early and late pregnancy.

Early pregnancy

The clinician requires information about the developing fetus in early pregnancy to assist him in the management of certain problems.

1. Threatened abortion.
2. Missed abortion.
3. Recurrent abortion.

The reader will find full accounts of the problem of abortion in gynaecological textbooks, and details given here will be limited.

In threatened abortion the pregnant woman experiences painless uterine bleeding. Occasionally there is some backache, or lower abdominal discomfort, but these are not marked features, as compared with inevitable abortion where the uterus contracts to expel the conceptus, and pain usually accompanies the bleeding.

About 30 per cent of women who present with threatened abortion, will inevitably abort. Most of the remainder will continue their pregnancies beyond 28 weeks. Although opinions vary, there has been no convincing evidence linking threatened abortion and congenital abnormality. (It must be remembered that there is a high incidence of fetal malformation in *inevitable* abortion, and this is usually quoted as 50–80 per cent.)

Although one can reassure the patient that she has no greater chance of producing an abnormal baby, nevertheless the perinatal mortality is 2·4 times greater than normal, presumably because some degree of placental damage has occurred.

A few cases of threatened abortion will become *missed*

abortions. Here the fetus dies but is not expelled. The usual presentation is that of a threatened abortion, the symptoms of which disappear and it later becomes clear that the uterus is not enlarging. Hypofibrinogenaemia is a possible sequel of this condition, but not usually until the fetus has been dead for four weeks.

A woman who has three consecutive pregnancies ending in abortion is said to be a recurrent (or habitual) aborter. Considerable pessimism has been expressed as to the outcome in these cases, but probably 60–80 per cent of such women, in their next pregnancy, will go past 28 weeks, often to term, albeit with an increased perinatal mortality.

CLINICAL ASSESSMENT

Bimanual pelvic examination in the first twelve weeks of pregnancy gives a very accurate estimate of the size of the growing uterus. The uterus will be smaller than expected for the length of the pregnancy in incomplete and missed abortion. In the former, examination of the cervix, carried out at the same time, will show it to be dilated, whereas in cases of threatened abortion, and usually in missed abortion, it is closed.

Examination of the cervix is also important where there is a history of second trimester abortion, where cervical incompetence is suspected. Dilatation of the cervix and subsequent abortion may be prevented by an encircling suture, e.g. the Shirodkar suture, and success achieved in about 70 per cent of cases.

From about 10 weeks of pregnancy the movement of the fetal blood can be detected by instruments, e.g. 'Doptone'* or 'Sonicaid'* which utilize the Doppler effect. An audible signal is produced which pulses at the same rate as the fetal heart beat. The information is clearly of great use in cases where it is difficult to decide whether the pregnancy is alive or not. The necessary equipment is simple to use, inexpensive, and portable.

*Registered trade marks.

ESTIMATION OF HUMAN CHORIONIC GONADOTROPHIN (H.C.G.)

H.C.G. is first detectable in the maternal urine at the fifth week of amenorrhoea. Its production by the trophoblast (probably the cytotrophoblast) gradually increases to a peak between the eighth and eleventh week, after which there is a progressive fall until the fifteenth week. A low level is maintained throughout the remainder of pregnancy. It is usually measured by one of the haemagglutination-inhibition pregnancy tests, e.g. Preparin, Pregnosticon, Gravindex, etc. using urine in a series of dilutions.

It has been shown in cases of threatened abortion in which the H.C.G. levels are low for the stage of the pregnancy, there exists a greatly increased chance that the pregnancy will proceed to an inevitable abortion. In cases where the levels are normal the prognosis is good. In missed abortion the levels are very low. In cases with a history of recurrent abortion, the wellbeing of the pregnancy (and response to any treatment) can be monitored by repeated H.C.G. estimations. Abnormally high levels may indicate hydatidiform mole. Multiple pregnancy may also be associated with higher-than-normal levels.

TABLE 3.4. *The normal excretory levels found in early morning urine specimens.* (*After Wide.*)

Weeks of pregnancy	*Mean value* (H.C.G.I.U/litre)	*Range* (H.C.G.I.U / litre)
6	8,000	1,000–40,000
7	40,000	15,000–100,000
8	80,000	40,000–200,000
9–10	100,000	40,000–400,000
11–12	90,000	40,000–300,000
13–15	70,000	20,000–250,000
16–17	30,000	15,000–100,000
20	25,000	10,000–50,000
24	20,000	10,000–50,000
32	20,000	2,500–50,000

The normal excretory levels found in early morning urine specimens are shown in Table 3.4.

VAGINAL CYTOLOGY

Progestogen therapy is used for a large number of cases of threatened abortion and in pregnant women with a history of abortion. In most cases this is unnecessary as only a small number of abortions are due to progesterone deficiency.

Examination of a stained smear taken from the lateral vaginal wall by means of a spatula, can provide some indication of the presence or absence of progesterone deficiency. Deficiency is associated with a decrease in the number of navicular cells and cell clusters become smaller. The number of superficial cells increases, and can be recognized by their pyknotic nuclei. These can be counted and expressed as the karyopyknotic index (K.P.I.) which is raised where there is progesterone deficiency.

In cases where vaginal cytology shows progesterone deficiency, the administration of progestogens may restore the cytology to normal.

The therapy can consist of weekly injections of progesterone derivatives, e.g. 17α-hydroxyprogesterone caproate 250 mg or hydrogesterone 15 mg, daily by mouth until 18 weeks. Virilization of a female fetus is not likely to occur with these substances.

This form of investigation and treatment is in common use, but its value, in terms of fetal salvage, has yet to be defined. The presence of endometrial cells indicates that the abortion has become inevitable. Changes in vaginal cytology in missed abortion are less helpful.

ESTIMATION OF HUMAN PLACENTAL LACTOGEN

This is another hormone product of the placenta, and is elaborated in the syncytiotrophoblast. It is becoming known also as 'human chorionic somatomammotrophin' (H.C.S.). It is measured in plasma samples by means of a radioimmunoassay, and has been found to be present in increasing amounts to term. These are usually expressed as immunoradio-assayable H.C.S. (I.R.H.C.S.) ng per ml and these levels are shown in Fig. 3.1.

FIG. 3.1. *I.R.H.C.S. levels in normal pregnancy.* (*After Ganezzani et al.*)

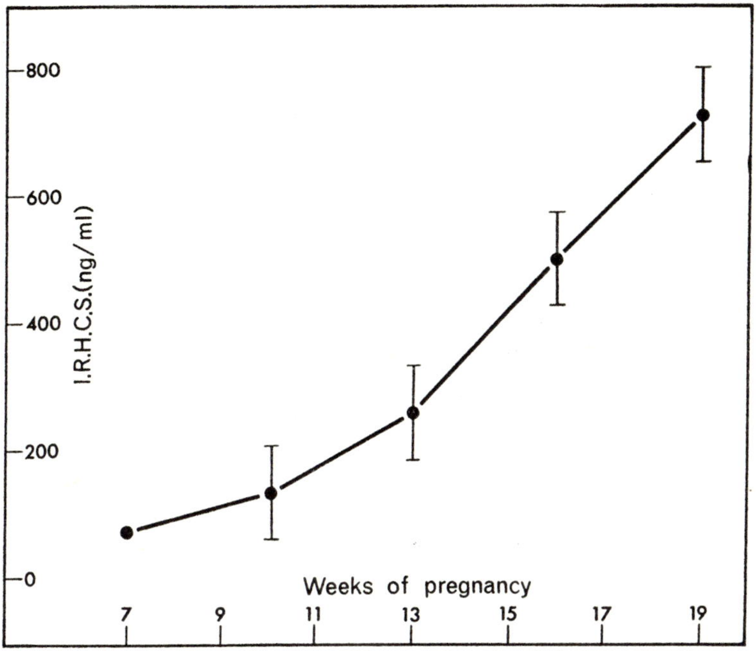

As in H.C.G. estimations, lower amounts are found where the prognosis in cases of threatened abortion is poor.

Late pregnancy

OESTROGEN EXCRETION

During recent years, it has become generally accepted that estimation of oestrogens in the maternal urine is the most accurate and helpful method available for the assessment of placental function and fetal wellbeing. Oestrogen excretion has been studied by many workers and a definite relationship has been established between low levels of excretion and increased perinatal mortality and morbidity, in the conditions listed in the introduction to this chapter.

Oestrogen synthesis. In order to produce oestrogens, mainly oestriol, certain metabolic pathways in the fetus are required. The precursors of steroid hormones, e.g. acetate, cholesterol, and pregnenolone need to be 'processed' in the fetus before being returned to the placenta to be converted to oestriol by aromatization.

FIG. 3.2. *The production of oestriol from the precursor pregnenolone.*

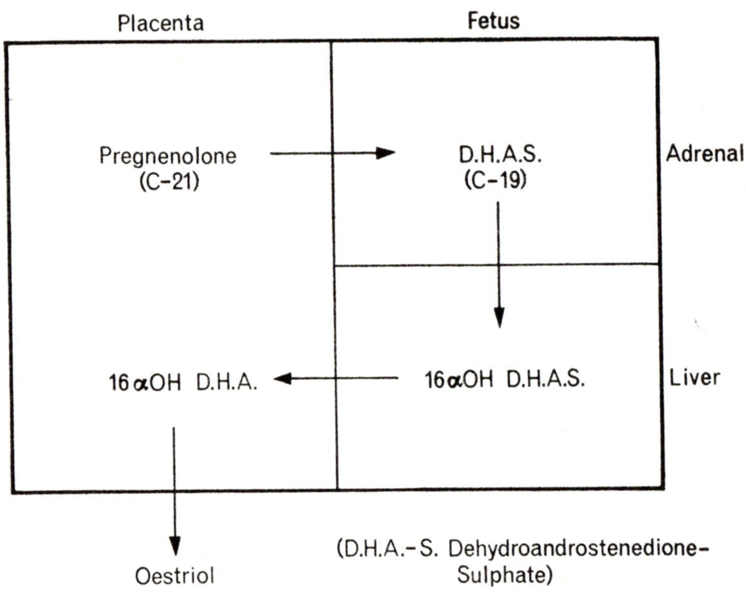

Fig. 3.2 summarizes the production of oestriol from the precursor pregnenolone, which is produced by the placenta.

It can be seen that the placenta not only lacks enzyme systems to convert C-21 steroids (such as progesterone and pregnenolone) to C-19 steroids (D.H.A. or androstenedione), but also the 16α-hydroxylase, both of which systems are present in the fetus. Thus, the production of oestriol is a function of the feto-placental unit as a whole, and clearly oestriol assay is of considerable clinical value in that it provides information about both the placenta *and* the fetus. Also the human fetal adrenal gland is an active centre of steroid production, and is relatively much larger than the adult gland. This hypertrophy is mainly due to the 'fetal-zone', a reticular area which involutes soon after birth. Where there is reduction of adrenal activity, as in anencephalics, or as a consequence of administration of cortisone or its analogues to the mother, there is a decrease in oestrogen production.

There are three principal fractions which collectively are called 'oestrogens'. Oestriol is by far the largest, and in late pregnancy is 90 per cent of the total. The other fractions, oestrone and oestradiol, are produced by the placenta from D.H.A. and androstenedione, and it has been shown also that 50 per cent of the production of these two oestrogens is from precursors formed in the maternal adrenal glands.

It is usual in clinical practice to measure only the oestriol fraction. On the other hand, as oestriol is present in such greater amounts than the other two, measurement of 'total oestrogens' although carried out by less refined techniques, is probably just as reliable.

Methods of assay. Although considerable expertise, time, and good laboratory services are required, an increasing number of maternity units in the U.K. are now provided with facilities for oestrogen assay. Quicker methods are now being developed involving automation, and gas-liquid chromatography. Details of the techniques in use lie outside the scope of this book.

At the present time estimation of urinary oestrogens is the standard method. Urine collected through 24 hours is used. Difficulties can be encountered in the collection of the specimens, and the patient must understand clearly what is required, so that the final specimen is quite complete. A suitable procedure would be to commence the 24 hours in the morning after emptying the bladder of the overnight urine. All urine passed is saved in a suitable bottle, and the collection is completed the following morning by the addition of the overnight urine voided after waking. The estimation is usually expressed as milligrams of oestriol (or total oestrogens) per 24 hours. It is

4

important that the laboratory indicate the volume of urine received. Where serial estimations are performed, marked variation in the urine volumes, will cast doubt upon the validity of the results.

Completeness of the urine collection can be confirmed by measuring the creatinine content of the specimen. The mean creatinine excretion in 24 hours is 1·35 g with a range of 0·29 to 2·9 g. A correction equation has been suggested, viz.

$$\frac{\text{oestriol (mg)}}{\text{creatinine (g)}} \times 1{\cdot}35$$

Certain drugs affect oestrogen levels, apart from corticosteroid therapy already mentioned. The urinary antiseptic Mandelamine has a marked effect and laxatives containing phenophthalein or 1 : 8 dihydroxyanthraquinone can interfere where colorimetric techniques are used.

It is likely that gas-liquid chromatography will be used on blood and liquor amnii samples in the future, thus allowing quicker results and assessment of the state of the feto-placental unit at more specific times.

Normal oestrogen levels. Excretion of oestrogens increases during normal pregnancy and the range of normal values is shown in Fig. 3.3. This shows levels at the various stages of gestation, and would be a suitable chart for plotting the results of serial estimations. It will be obvious that it is necessary to be certain of the length of gestation. Isolated readings are of limited value and repeated estimations are infinitely preferable.

Despite the obvious advantages of oestriol measurements in maternal blood, such techniques have not come into common clinical usage. There is considerable variation in published figures for levels in blood and liquor amnii.

ABNORMAL PREGNANCY

Serial oestriol estimations in the maternal urine give the clinician the best information about the potential of the fetus to survive. They are of particular value where 'placental insufficiency' is suspected, e.g. pre-eclampsia, poor obstetric history, retarded intrauterine growth etc. It must be em-

FIG. 3.3 *Urinary oestrogen levels in urine during late pregnancy.*

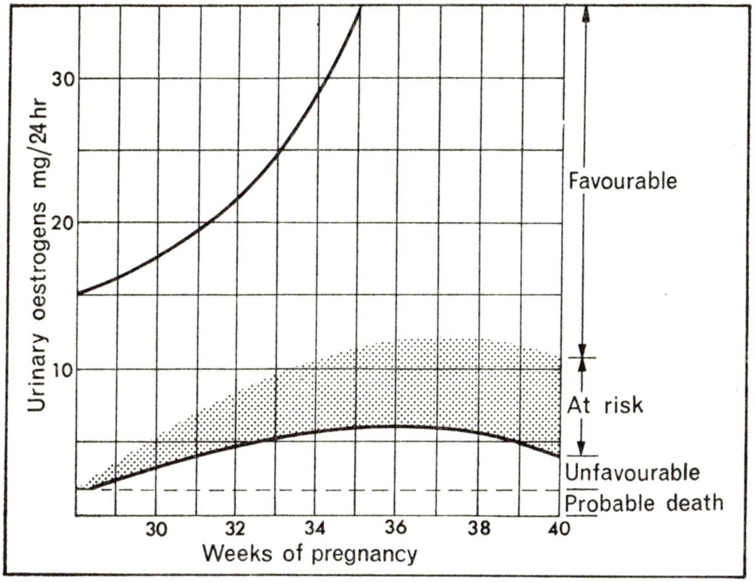

phasized that these estimations must be assessed in conjunction with careful clinical observations, as well as with the results of other placental function tests. Indeed, it is clinical examination of the pregnant woman that must give the first clue to there being something amiss. However, intrauterine death may occur in apparently normal pregnancies, and there is certainly a case for routine estimations of oestrogen levels in whole obstetric populations, and not just selected cases as at present. The advent of rapid measurements on maternal blood will help to bring this about.

Maternal hypertension. In hypertension there is reduced placental blood flow. This may produce hypoxia in the fetus, and may also retard intrauterine growth. The effects are usually proportional to the severity of the disease, and oestrogen levels reflect this severity. Levels do not seem to be lowered before the onset of pre-eclampsia. The trends of the levels are of great assistance in deciding when to deliver the baby, particularly in cases of early pre-eclampsia, e.g. 30–34 weeks where obviously the delivery later of a more mature infant is desirable. Oestrogen assays repeated once or twice weekly can reassure the clinician that all is well, or indicate that the fetus is in jeopardy, and therefore better off *ex utero*.

Retarded intrauterine growth. The 'light-for-dates' baby has been defined elsewhere in this book as have the hazards associated with the condition. Apart from the risk of subsequent morbidity, the still-birth and neonatal death rates are eight times those for normal birth weight babies of the same gestational age. Although it is the clinician who first suspects the condition, clinical assessment is notoriously unreliable. Serial oestrogen estimations can establish the diagnosis, and help him to decide the best time for early delivery. When fetal growth is retarded, oestrogen excretion is diminished in 90 per cent of cases.

Poor obstetric history. Serial studies are carried out in pregnant women where there has been a previous unexplained still-birth, previous 'light-for-dates' baby, history of unexplained fetal hypoxia, or placental insufficiency, in the hope of avoiding a further tragedy.

The clinician can be reassured that the pregnancy is progressing satisfactorily if the levels are normal. Conversely he may be given a timely warning of impending danger.

Prolonged pregnancy. There is usually no hazard to the fetus when a normal pregnancy is prolonged until 14 days past term. After this there is a greater risk of fetal death and the perinatal mortality at 42 weeks is twice that between 38 and 41 weeks. Most obstetricians perform induction of labour at this time, or even earlier, e.g. at 10 days post-term, and placental function tests are not carried out. Still-birth occurs rarely between term and 42 weeks in a completely normal pregnancy. It is possible that routine oestrogen level screening will select such cases, but until this becomes freely available observations of weight and girth, discussed elsewhere in this chapter, are probably of more value.

Antepartum haemorrhage. Serial oestrogen levels are of great value in assessing progress where an antepartum haemorrhage has occurred, and where placental damage may have been sustained. Weekly or bi-weekly measurements whilst the patient is awaiting the customary 'examination-under-anaesthetic: ? Caesarean section' should be made.

Diabetic pregnancy. Estimations are of doubtful value in the management of the diabetic pregnancy, except possibly where pre-eclampsia has developed, or where there is suspected retarded fetal growth.

Rhesus iso-immunization. The levels may be normal or high even where the fetus is severely affected, and are therefore of no value in this condition.

HEAT STABLE ALKALINE PHOSPHATASE (H.S.A.P.)

There is a fraction of the enzyme alkaline phosphatase which is present in the serum of pregnant women which appears to be produced on the maternal side of the placenta. It can be distinguished from non-placental phosphatases because it is heat-stable. Other phosphatases are inactivated at 56 °C. In order to avoid misleading results heating the serum to 65 °C is recommended. Methods of measurement are much simpler than for hormone assays. They are carried out on samples of serum, and results are obtained very quickly.

In pregnancy there is a normal rise as pregnancy progresses as shown in Fig. 3.4. Placental dysfunction has been shown to produce an abnormal rise above the normal scatter. Less frequently, a low amount has been associated with a failing placenta.

The method is undergoing enthusiastic evaluation at the present time in many departments because it is relatively easy to perform, and can be used frequently, e.g. daily if necessary. However, although abnormally high and abnormally low values are found associated with placental insufficiency, too many such cases have normal levels. It has been suggested that in only one-third of cases of placental insufficiency are H.S.A.P. levels abnormal.

FIG. 3.4. *Heat stable alkaline phosphatase levels in late pregnancy. The dots represent tests at 56 °C and the solid lines give the normal range at 65 °C.* (*After Hunter, and Curzen and Morris.*)

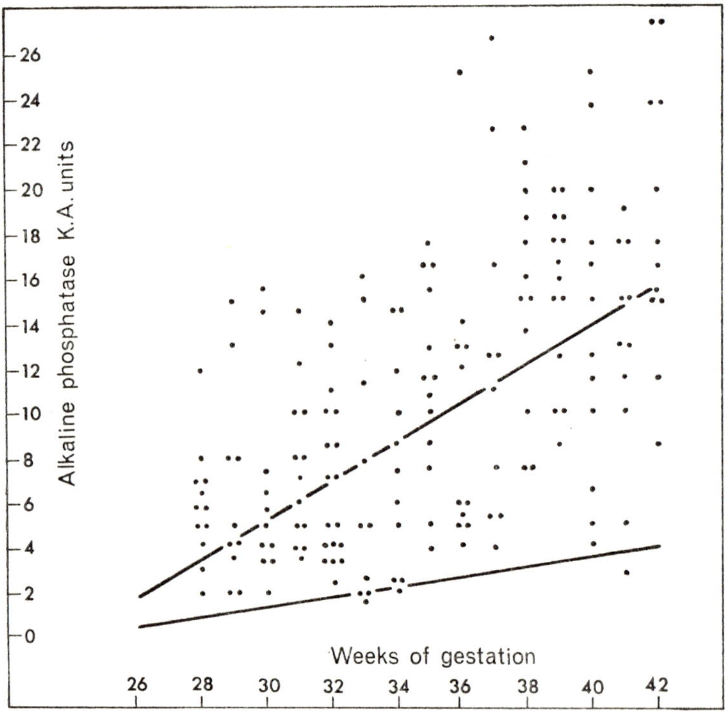

ESTIMATION OF HUMAN PLACENTAL LACTOGEN (H.P.L.)

This hormone, produced by the syncytiotrophoblast is currently under evaluation as an indicator of placental function. It has lactogenic activity and has immunological and biological resemblance to human growth hormone. Because of these observations, the name 'human chorionic somato-mammotrophin' (H.C.S.) has been regarded as more appropriate.

It is secreted mainly into the maternal circulation, and is present in levels higher than any other protein hormone. Small amounts only are found in cord blood. There is a rapid turnover, and it is measured in maternal serum by a radio-immunoassay technique, mentioned earlier in this chapter.

The normal range of levels is shown in Fig. 3.5.

Good correlation has been found between H.P.L. levels and

FIG. 3.5. *Normal levels of H.P.L.* (*After Saxena et al.*)

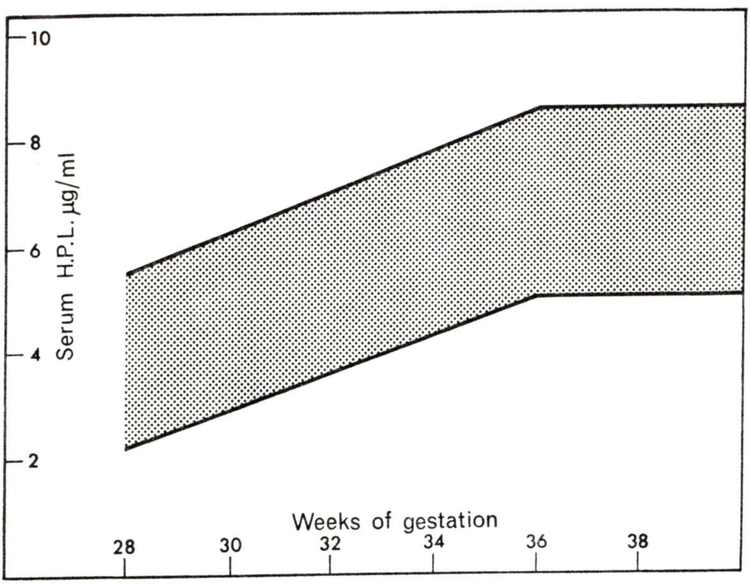

placental weight, and it would appear to be index of the placental function only, in contrast to oestrogens, whose metabolism involves the fetus.

Moreover, it has been shown to be of great practical value in the management of high risk pregnancies, particularly where placental insufficiency is suspected, and in the 'light-for-dates' baby. Low or diminishing levels are found in these conditions. High levels are found in diabetic pregnancy and multiple pregnancy.

As elaboration of this hormone appears to be totally within the placenta, estimations of it cannot be said to reflect changes in the feto-placental unit as a whole. Indeed death of the fetus may not alter the serum levels. Despite these experiences correlation has been claimed between H.P.L. and oestriol levels.

Nevertheless, the rapid accurate laboratory measurement of H.P.L. appears to have considerable clinical value, but it is unlikely to replace oestrogen estimations in obstetric practice, at the present time.

PROGESTERONE AND PREGNANEDIOL

Progesterone can be reliably measured in blood, but such estimations are not of great clinical value as an indicator of placental function. Pregnanediol is an end product, and can be measured in maternal urine in a 24-hour specimen.

After considerable initial enthusiasm, it is clear that urinary pregnanediol estimations have not proved very useful in clinical practice. This is largely due to the great variation in excretion patterns.

It is of great interest to note that, until recently, it was thought that the fetus played no part in the production of pregnanediol. It has been shown that the fetus plays a minor role, probably contributing up to 20 per cent of the steroid in maternal urine.

INCREASE IN WEIGHT AND GIRTH

Despite the pre-occupation with complex biochemical tests of placental function, it has been recognized for many years that simple observations of maternal weight and girth changes are of considerable value in assessing fetal wellbeing. It has been noted for some time that where placental insufficiency exists, the normal diminution in the liquor amnii near term may commence earlier. This would result in static or falling maternal girth. Similarly, in such situations the placenta may produce less oestrogen and progesterone, and there will be static or falling maternal weight due to reduced fluid retention.

These changes were noted to be more pronounced where maternal hypertension existed – notably in pre-eclampsia – and form an interesting contrast with the efforts to *prevent* excessive weight gain in our ante-natal clinics, to the extent of strict diet, salt restriction etc.

Weight measurement. Standardization of clinic scales appears impossible but checking their accuracy is not. The patients should wear a standard gown, and be weighed at about the same time of day at each visit. Sustained failure to gain weight, or sustained loss of one pound or more, particularly after 34 weeks, are significant.

Girth measurement. This is much more difficult than measuring weight. Different observers obtain widely differing measurements. Some measure the greatest obtainable abdominal circumference, but it is probably wiser to take a fixed point, e.g. the umbilicus, and find the smallest girth. Recordings should be to the nearest half inch, and should be made from 34 weeks onwards. Persistent failure to increase in girth, or persistent diminution of one inch or more, is significant.

One of the great difficulties in obtaining a meaningful series of these observations is due to the practice of 'shared' ante-natal care, e.g. between consultant and general practitioner. Observer and instrument differences are frequent. It is probably wiser if the clinician responsible for delivery undertakes all the ante-natal care in the later weeks of the pregnancy including after term.

Results. In a recent important study (some of the results are tabulated in Table 3.5), it has been shown that there was a significant difference in weight gain between pregnancies producing 'light-for-dates' babies and those producing normal birth weight babies. This difference was more marked after 34 weeks.

TABLE 3.5. *Difference in weight gain for pregnancies producing normal birth weight babies and 'light-for-dates' babies.* (*After Elder et al.*)

Baby	Weekly weight gain (lbs) *To 34 weeks*	*34 weeks to term*	*% patients static or falling weight 34 weeks to term*	*% patients static or falling girth 34 weeks to term*
'Light-for-dates'	0·79	0·40	58·8%	76·7%
Normal birth weight	0·86	0·68	21·5%	48%

The same study revealed an increased incidence of fetal distress in normal birth weight babies where there was weight loss after term. This method is clearly of value in the management of prolonged pregnancy, to guide the clinician in deciding if and when labour should be induced.

These observations have their greatest value in the hypertensive patient, but there is good reason why all pregnant women should be monitored in this way.

AMNIOSCOPY

Meconium-staining of the liquor amnii has been the subject of considerable controversy. Classically it is a sign of fetal 'distress', i.e. hypoxia, and has been, by some workers, associated with an increased perinatal mortality and increased incidence of neonatal asphyxia. Its value as a danger sign has probably been overstated, and some authorities have suggested it is merely a reflex mechanism due to distension of the fetal colon; others, that it is pure chance defaecation by a normal fetus.

The perinatal mortality where no fetal distress is present, is about 2 per cent. In cases with meconium-staining of the liquor but a normal fetal heart rate, it is 4–7 per cent. Where the fetal heart rate has become abnormal also, the mortality is considerably raised, possibly as much as 20 per cent. In addition, increased morbidity and mortality must be expected when meconium is present in the liquor of patients with *other* factors, e.g. pre-eclampsia, prolonged pregnancy etc.

Amnioscopy offers a way of detecting meconium in the liquor before the membranes are ruptured and before labour commences. The volume of liquor can also be roughly assessed by the amount of forewaters present. Oligohydramnios may be a warning of antepartum hypoxia.

The technique is simple and can be performed on outpatients in five to six minutes. It is usually performed with the patient in lithotomy position. Amnioscopes are tapered metal tubes, and there are different sizes, based on the diameter of the cervical end, for different degrees of cervical dilatation. There is a light source, the liquor being visualized by reflected light from the fetal skull. The procedure causes little discomfort and may be repeated frequently. Accidental rupture of the membranes occurs in 2–3 per cent of patients, and one must also be aware of the unexpected placenta praevia. Bleeding from separation of the membranes from the lower segment, following the examination, is very frequent, but usually stops spontaneously. Infection is rare.

Amnioscopy provides a way of monitoring the fetus which is at risk from progressive hypoxia, and guiding the clinician as to when to induce labour. It should remove the need for routine induction, e.g. at 42 weeks, for prolonged labour, at 38 weeks for pre-eclampsia etc. By this means the actual induction rate should be reduced and likewise the caesarean section rate, and this has been found by many workers. Whether there is a significant reduction in perinatal mortality is still in some dispute.

The early appearance of meconium in the liquor, will alert the clinician to monitor the fetus even more closely, during the ensuing labour.

ULTRA-SOUND

Where the placental function is abnormal, one would certainly expect fetal growth to be affected. Direct estimation of this is possible, by measurement of the biparietal diameter of the fetal skull by ultrasonic scanning. Repeated weekly examinations can be made, and growth rate measured.

It has been suggested that where the rate of increase in size of the biparietal diameter is *a.* less than 0·17 cm per week, then 70·4 per cent of such cases will be 'light-for-dates', *b.* more than 0·17 cm per week, then 69·1 per cent of such cases will be of normal birth weight.

It has also been shown that if the diameter is 8·5 cm or more, then 91 per cent of such babies will be 2,500 g or over, in weight.

Expensive equipment is required, plus skilled help, but clearly this is a valuable aid in the management of the 'at risk' fetus.

In high intensities, ultra-sound has been shown to produce chromosome breakages in cell nuclei, and to alter nerve conduction in experimental preparations. No such adverse effects have been noted in clinical usage, but the matter is continuously under review. (See also chapter 7.)

RADIOACTIVE SELENOMETHIONINE UPTAKE

Amino-acids are taken up by the fetus from the maternal circulation via the placenta. A method of assessing fetal growth by measuring the amount of an amino-acid which is transferred to the fetus over a short period of time has been described. The techniques involved are not difficult and the apparatus required is not elaborate or expensive.

Two microcuries of ^{75}Se-Selenomethionine are injected intravenously and the gamma rays emitted are detected simultaneously over the uterus and the sternum by highly sensitive sodium iodine crystal detectors. The count over the sternum is necessary to correct for body build differences between patients. The count rate over the uterus is divided by the count rate over the sternum (measured at the same time), called the uptake ratio.

The uptake ratio is made 15 minutes following the injection and again after one to three days. There appears to be good correlation between these readings and therefore the first ratio obtained is reliable. In practice, ratios of 0·5–0·6 at 15 minutes, and 0·6–0·7 at a second reading indicate normal uptake. The placenta appears able to extract the amino-acid from maternal blood, and therefore normal fetal growth is assumed. The radiation dose is small, viz. 13 millirads to mother, and 20 millirads to the fetus. In comparison, the amounts from a plain X-ray of the maternal abdomen are 367 and 723 respectively.

DEHYDROEPIANDROSTERONE-SULPHATE (D.H.A.S.) LOAD TEST

The D.H.A.S. load test involves the administration of this oestriol precursor to the mother and measuring the increase in oestriol excretion produced.

A two-hour sample of urine is collected and the basal oestriol excretion is estimated. An injection of 30 mg D.H.A.S. is given and urinary oestriols measured at two-hourly intervals. In normal pregnancy maximum excretion occurs after two hours; with slightly reduced placental function after four hours; with more severely affected function, after six hours.

VAGINAL CYTOLOGY

One would expect the epithelium of the vagina to reflect hormonal changes. Thus if 'placental insufficiency' occurs, cytological examination of a stained smear of vaginal squames should demonstrate certain changes, which may be helpful.

Smears are collected with a spatula, either from the lateral vaginal wall or the posterior fornix, and are stained by Papanicolaou's, or Shorr's method.

This technique has never been popular in this country, despite several distinguished protagonists. Even though the collection and processing of material is simple, the interpretation of it has not been standardized. The reader is referred to several sources, but will find differing cytological criteria laid down, and much will depend on the enthusiasm of the clinician for the method.

References and guides to further reading

ALEEM, F. A. et al. (1969). 'Clinical significance of the amniotic fluid oestriol level', *J. Obstet. Gynaec. Br. Commonw.*, **76**, 200.

BAIRD, D. T. (1968). 'A method for the measurement of estrone and estradiol – 17β in peripheral human blood and other biological fluids using 35s Pipsyl Chloride', *J. Clin. Endocr.*, **28**, 244.

BEISCHER, N. A. et al. (1968). 'The incidence and significance of low oestriol excretion in an obstetric population', *J. Obstet. Gynaec. Br. Commonw.*, **75**, 1024.

BROWN, J. B. et al. (1957). 'An additional purification strip for a method for estimating oestriol, oestrone and oestradiol 17β in human urine', *J. Endocr.*, **16**, 49.

VAN DER CRABBEN, H. et al. (1970). 'A list of placental function using the oestrogen precussor dehydroepiandrosterone sulphate', Proceedings of Second European Congress of Perinatal Medicine, London.

COYLE, M. G., and BROWN, J. B. (1963). 'Urinary excretion of oestriol during pregnancy', *J. Obstet. Gynaec. Br. Commonw.*, **70**, 225.

DICKEY, R. P. et al. (1966). 'Diurnal excretion of estrogen and creatinine during pregnancy', *Am. J. Obstet. Gynaec.*, **94**, 591.

ENEIN, M. A. A., and SHARMAN, A. (1967). 'Immuno-assay of human chorionic gonadotrophin in threatened abortion', *J. Obstet. Gynaec. Br. Commonw.*, **74**, 583.

ELDER, M. G. et al. (1970). 'Maternal weight and girth changes in late pregnancy and the diagnosis of placental insufficiency', *J. Obstet. Gynaec. Br. Commonw.*, **77**, 481.

GARROW, J. S., and DOUGLAS, C. P. (1968). 'A rapid method for assessing intrauterine growth by radioactive selenomethionine', *J. Obstet. Gynaec. Br. Commonw.*, **75**, 1034.

GENAZZANI, A. R. 'Radioimmunoassay of human chorionic somatotrophin (HCS or HPL)', *Acta endocr.* (*Kbh*), Suppl. 138, 7.

—— et al. (1969). 'Use of human-placental-lactogen radioimmunoassay to predict outcome in cases of threatened abortion', *Lancet*, **2**, 1385.

HENRY, G. R. (1970). 'Amnioscopy', *Brit. J. Hosp. Med.*, **3**, 516.

HUNTER, R. J. (1969). 'Serum heat stable alkaline phosphatase: an index of placental function', *J. Obstet. Gynaec. Br. Commonw.*, **76**, 1057.

ITTRICH, G. (1960). 'Studies on the extraction of red Kober dyes by organic solvents for the determination of urinary oestrogens', *Acta endocr.* (*Kbh*), **35**, 34.

KLOPPER, A. (1969). 'Foetus and Placenta' (Ed. Klopper and Diczfalusy), Blackwell Scientific Publications, Oxford and Edinburgh, 471.

LEETON, J. et al. (1967). 'Vaginal Cytohormonal studies in late abnormal pregnancy', *Acta cytol.* (*Balt.*), **11**, 410.

MICHIE, E. A., and LIVINGSTONE, J. R. B. (1969). 'Oestriol concentration in amniotic fluid', *Acta endocr.*, **61**, 329.

OAKEY, R. E. et al. (1967). 'The rapid estimation of oestrogens in pregnancy to monitor foetal risk', *Clinica. Chim. Acta*, **15**, 35.

SALING, E. (1968). 'Foetal and Neonatal Hypoxia in relation to Clinical Obstetric Practice', Edward Arnold, London.

SAXENA, B. N. et al. (1969). 'Serum placental lactogen (HPL) levels as an index of placental function', *New England J. Med.*, **281,** 225.

SPELLACY, W. N. et al. (1967). 'Human placental lactogen levels as a measure of placental function', *Am. J. Obstet. Gynaec.*, **97,** 560.

WACHTEL, E. G. (1964). 'Exfolicitive Cytology in Gynaeological Practice', Butterworth, London.

WATNEY, P. J. M. *et al.* (1970). 'The relative usefulness of methods of assessing placental function', *J. Obstet. Gynaec. Br. Commonw.*, **77,** 301.

WILCOCKS, J. et al. (1967). 'Intrauterine growth assessed by ultrasonic foetal cephalometry', *J. Obstet. Gynaec. Br. Commonw.*, **74,** 639.

WIDE, L. (1962). 'Immunological method for the assay of human chorionic gonadotrophin', *Acta endo.* (*Kbh*), 41 (Suppl. 70).

WOOD, C. et al. (1961). 'Vaginal cytology in pregnancy', *J. Obstet Gynaec. Br. Commonw.*, **68,** 778.

WOTIZ, H. H. et al. (1962). 'Studies in steroid metabolism. XI. Gas chromatographic determination of estrogens in human pregnancy urine', *Analyt. Biochem.*, **3,** 97.

CHAPTER 4

ESTIMATION OF LENGTH OF GESTATION

The clinician frequently needs to know, as accurately as possible, the length of gestation to help him manage certain obstetric problems. These almost all involve the termination of a pregnancy, by induction of labour or caesarean section, to minimize the hazard to the fetus and/or mother produced by the particular obstetric problem. On the other hand, such interference should be timely and not add to the already too high incidence of premature labours.

The obstetric problems where planned delivery might be indicated are as follows:

1. Pre-eclampsia.
2. Essential hypertension.
3. Hypertensive renal disease.
4. Rhesus iso-immunization.
5. Diabetes mellitus.
6. 'Light-for-dates' pregnancies.
7. Previous late unexpected still-birth due to placental insufficiency.
8. Evidence of antepartum placental insufficiency.
9. Borderline disproportion.
10. Antepartum haemorrhage.

11. Breech presentation.
12. Advanced maternal age.
13. Elective caesarean section for any reason.
14. Previous caesarean section.
15. Prolonged pregnancy.

Clearly it is important that the baby should be as mature as possible, taking into account the hazards of the intrauterine environment. Equally, the dangers of removing an immature fetus from one relatively dangerous situation and placing it in another, cannot be overstated. For example, to induce labour in a case of pre-eclampsia at presumed 39 weeks and then to deliver the mother of a 35-week baby, who then dies of respiratory distress syndrome, would be an avoidable iatrogenic tragedy. As can be seen from Fig. 4.1 the perinatal mortality ratio, even at 38 weeks, is double that at 39 weeks. It has also been shown that the still-birth and neonatal death rates in 'light-for-dates' babies is eight times that for babies of normal weight, for their period of gestation.

The time-honoured method of calculating the expected date of delivery (E.D.D.) in a particular pregnancy is based on Naegele's rule of 1812, which measures the menstruation-delivery interval. The E.D.D. is found by adding 7 days and 9 months to the date of the first day of the last normal menstrual period (L.N.M.P.). It would be more accurate to measure the fertilization-delivery interval, but clearly this would be more difficult and require sophisticated and expensive techniques, so accuracy is sacrificed for convenience. To be certain of the L.N.M.P. is often difficult for the reasons summarized:

1. Failure by the pregnant woman to note or remember the date of the L.N.M.P.
2. Irregular or prolonged menstrual cycles.
3. Early bleeding, threatened abortion, decidual and implanation bleeds.
4. The contraceptive pill.
5. The unreliability of clinical assessment unless made in early pregnancy.

It is unfortunately very common for women to be unsure of

FIG. 4.1. *Survey mortality ratio (M) at weekly gestations near term in non-toxaemic, toxaemic, and all pregnancies. (Adapted from Butler and Bonham.)*

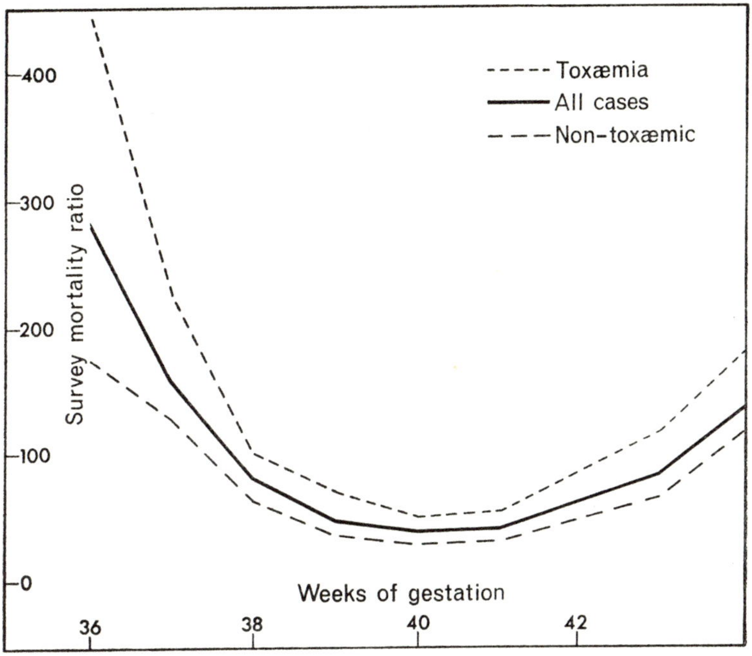

the date of their last menstrual period, and this, above all, produces clinical problems in the estimation of the length of gestation.

The contraceptive pill is becoming increasingly popular, and the withdrawal bleeding produced may be confused with actual menstruation. Following cessation of oral contraceptive administration variable intervals of amenorrhoea can occur and, should fertilization take place during this time, it may be extremely difficult to pinpoint the beginning of a pregnancy.

CLINICAL ASSESSMENT

The clinician can be most accurate in his estimate of length of pregnancy in the first trimester. During the first twelve weeks a bimanual pelvic examination is essential, and particularly so if there is any doubt concerning the date of the last normal menstrual period. The findings at this time can influence management at the other end of the pregnancy. Alteration in the rate of intrauterine growth can be observed early, and this is of value in the 'light-for-dates' baby. One is measuring actual uterine size, and the need for early bookings at ante-natal clinics cannot be overstressed. Later, abdominal examination is utilized. This relates the level of the uterine fundus to various anatomical points, viz. pubis, umbilicus, and xiphisternum (in either finger-breadths or centimetres). Fig. 4.2 shows the relationship of fundal height to length of gestation.

FIG. 4.2. *The relationship of fundal height to the length of gestation.*

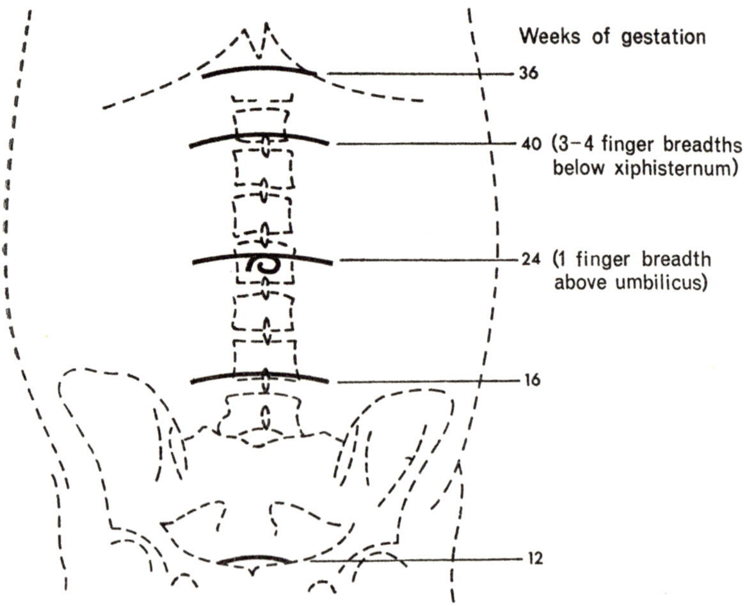

If one uses the finger-breadth method, the fundal height rises by roughly one finger-breadth each fortnight. The fundus is felt just above the symphysis pubis at 12 weeks, one finger-breadth above the umbilicus at 24 weeks, and at the xiphisternum at 36 weeks. In the primigravida one would expect at term, because of engagement of the head, that the fundus be 3 or 4 finger-breadths below the xiphisternum. Observer-differences are frequent and tend to occur at ante-natal clinics where patients are seen by several clinicians. After the first trimester, abdominal examination can give nothing more than a crude estimation, and the observer cannot expect to be more precise than to within 4 weeks of the actual gestational age by these methods. It must be clear that where the length of the pregnancy in weeks from the L.N.M.P. is in doubt, clinical problems may actually be created by the clinician himself. Unnecessary interference or delayed interference may result in perinatal mortality.

RADIOLOGY

An X-ray of the maternal abdomen, a prone view, allows visualization of the fetus. Certain features can be examined and an assessment of gestational age made. The criteria on which this assessment is based are imprecise, and not equally acceptable to all radiologists. The potential dangers of radiation are present, however slight the risk, and it is not possible to avoid irradiating fetal and maternal gonads.

The main criteria on which assessment of maturity is made are as follows:

1. Appearance of ossific centres in the knee and the feet.
2. Fat thickness.
3. General appearances.

Other criteria used are:

4. Length of femoral diaphysis.
5. Size of skull.

Ossific centres. The usually quoted times of appearance of the epiphyses of the knee joint are as follows:

a. lower femoral, 36 weeks,

b. upper tibial, 38 weeks.

The degree of development of these epiphyses is also taken

into account, and the radiologist can gauge whether the fetus is at, or past, term. Clearly the films must be of optimum quality, and standardized in exposure and processing. The tarsal cuboid ossific centre is considered by some radiologists to appear at 40 weeks, and by others at 36 weeks. It is usually less easy to see than the knee joint centres.

There is considerable biological variation in the appearance of these centres. They may not be symmetrically developed in the same fetus, and may be quite different in twins. Maternal diabetes and anencephaly are considered by some to accelerate their development, while retarded intrauterine growth and 'light-for-dates' syndromes may delay them.

Despite these variations, difference of opinion, and difficulties in visualization, e.g. overlying maternal bones, blurring due to fetal movement etc., the appearances of ossific centres remain the most popularly used parameter of fetal maturity.

Fat thickness. A well developed fat thickness over a fetal shoulder usually indicates a mature infant. In interpreting these radiological appearances it must be remembered that in diabetic and hydropic babies this layer may be excessively thick. Conversely it may be poorly developed in the 'light-for-dates' baby, and mislead the clinician into underestimating the length of gestation.

General appearances. The clinician can derive some help from the overall appearances, particularly the calcification of the skull and the length of the fetus, but these should never be used in isolation.

Length of femoral diaphysis. It has been claimed that from this measurement fetal size and age can be ascertained. However, the femora often appear foreshortened on the maternal abdominal view.

Size of skull. X-ray cephalometry has its protagonists. The fetal age is calculated from a suitable scattergraph showing skull diameter related to length of gestation. However, it requires two exposures and is less easy when the fetal head is below the pelvic brim.

This measurement can be carried out by ultrasonic techniques without the need for X-radiation exposure.

ULTRASONIC MEASUREMENT

Measurement of the fetal biparietal diameter by ultrasonic techniques relies on analysis of the echo produced by the fetal parietal bones and midline structures. Such measurements are accurate to within 0·1 cm.

Growth curves for biparietal diameters throughout pregnancy have been produced and indicate that the rate is not uniform throughout pregnancy. Ultrasonic measurements are possible from about the twentieth week onwards and serial measurements starting as early as possible are necessary because the rate of growth is more informative than the absolute size. This rate varies with the length of gestation and between 20 and 30 weeks has a mean value of 0·28 cm/week, but measurements should be plotted on a growth/gestational age chart such as that shown in Fig. 4.3. Where the growth rate is normal, especially based on measurements between the twentieth and thirtieth weeks, extrapolation can give an accurate prediction of E.D.D. in over 90 per cent of cases.

Expensive apparatus is required and also skilled technical assistance. As the most usual situation of doubtful length of gestation occurs towards the end of pregnancy, i.e. the last six weeks, this technique is of limited clinical value, unless employed from the middle trimester.

VAGINAL CYTOLOGY

The examination of a stained smear of vaginal cells has been used to predict the proximity of term. It has never been popular in the U.K. as a routine technique because descriptions and interpretations vary between authors. Smears may be classified into 'late pregnancy', 'near term', and 'term'. This is based on

FIG. 4.3. *Fetal biparietal diameter from 20–30 weeks.* (*Cambell, S. 1969. J. Obstet. Gynaec. Br. Commonw.*, 76, *603*.)

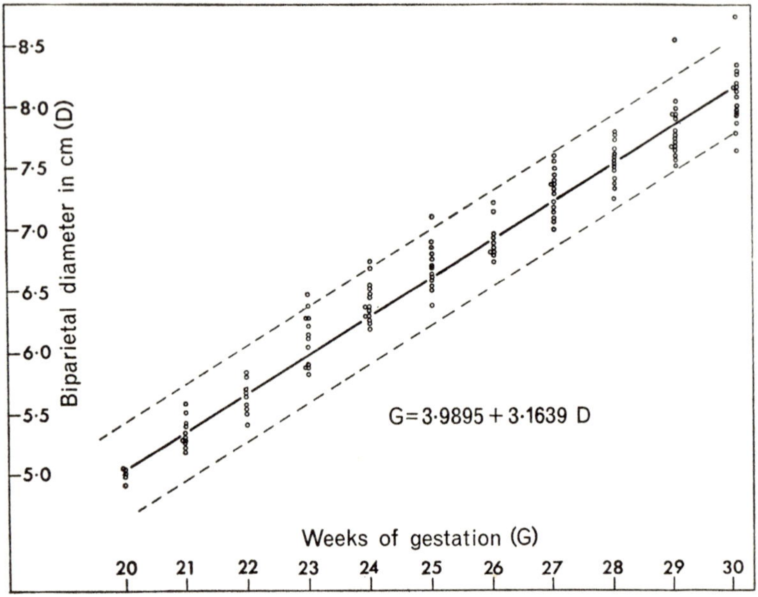

quantitative changes, e.g. a decrease in navicular cells, and an increase in superficial and intermediate squames, and leucocytes, towards term. These changes do occur but they are not regular enough to be of any great value to the clinician.

AMNIOTIC FLUID STUDIES

1. Biochemical.
2. Cytological.

These involve sampling of amniotic fluid by amniocentesis (for technique see appendix).

1. *Biochemical*

a. Creatinine. Concentrations increase steadily after 30 weeks. The most reliable level observed is 1·8 mg % when the fetus is almost certainly 36 weeks or more. It is sometimes abnormally high in diabetic pregnancies and appears to be helpful in 'light-for-dates' babies.

b. Bilirubin. The concentration of bilirubin in the amniotic fluid decreases as pregnancy advances. It is clearly no use in cases of blood group incompatibility. There is a wide scatter of values in relation to length of gestation and, despite some enthusiastic workers, measurement of bilirubin has not been shown to be of great value when used in isolation.

c. Osmolality. Total electrolyte concentrations fall during pregnancy and can be measured in milli-osmoles (mOs) per litre. This is based on freezing-point depression, and requires special elaborate apparatus. If the liquid osmolality is 250 mOs/litre or less, the fetus is 38 weeks or more.

d. Urea and proteins. Estimation of these in amniotic fluid has not been shown to be helpful in assessing length of gestation.

2. *Cytological*

The extremely simple method of straining liquor with Nile Blue Sulphate, and counting the orange and blue stained cells in a field of 200 or 500, has now become an almost standard procedure in late pregnancy where there is doubt about the length of the pregnancy. A drop of liquor and a drop of the stain are mixed on a slide, warmed gently, and examined under the low power objective. If the percentage of orange-stained cells is in excess of 40 per cent or if there is well-marked clumping of these cells, the fetus is 38 weeks or more. Sometimes when the fetus is past term, free fat globules are noted, but this is by no means consistent. The orange stained cells are believed to be sebaceous in origin and are present in small numbers before 38 weeks, but appear in profusion at this time. It is a useful test in the management of 'light-for-dates' babies as it appears to be unaffected by placental dysfunction disorders. The technique takes a few minutes only, and coupled with the relative safety of amniocentesis, provides a very helpful tool for the clinician.

VISUALIZATION OF THE VERNIX

If, following a trans-abdominal injection of the dye Ethiodan into the amniotic sac, an x-ray of the maternal abdomen is taken 8–24 hours later, the vernix caseosa, now radio-opaque, is visible on the film.

1. If the whole fetus is outlined, the pregnancy is less than 38 weeks.
2. If the outline is patchy over the limbs, trunk and abdomen, the fetus is 38–40 weeks.
3. If the outline has almost disappeared, the fetus is at term.

This method has been successfully combined with cytological examination. However, the answer to the clinical problem in a particular case, is delayed, maybe to the following day because of the time required for the vernix to take up the dye.

Conclusion

No absolutely accurate single method of assessing length of gestation is available to the clinician. Considering the non-availability of expensive equipment and the need for rapid information, probably the most useful combination of investigations would be a plain maternal abdominal X-ray followed if necessary by amniocentesis and Nile Blue Sulphate staining of the liquor. The X-ray would also show undiagnosed multiple pregnancy and unsuspected fetal abnormality. Many obstetricians now routinely request an X-ray of the maternal abdomen where induction of labour is indicated.

The really interesting question yet to be answered is whether these investigations measure actual length of gestation, biological maturity, or fitness to survive, and which of these is the most important.

References and guides to further reading

BROSENS, I., and GORDON, H. (1966). 'The estimation of maturity by cytological examination of the liquor amnii', *J. Obstet. Gynaec. Br. Commonw.*, **73**, 88.

—— —— and BAERT, A. (1969). 'Prediction of fetal maturity with combined cytological and radiological methods', *ibid.*, **76**, 20.

CAMPBELL, S. (1969). 'The prediction of fetal maturity by ultrasonic measurement of the biparietal diameter', *ibid.*, **76**, 603.

MANDELBAUM, B., and EVANS, T. N. (1969). 'Life in the amniotic fluid', *Am. J. Obstet. Gynec.*, **104**, 365.

RUSSELL, J. G. B. (1969). 'Radiological assessment of fetal maturity', *J. Obstet. Gynaec. Br. Commonw.*, **76**, 208.

CHAPTER 5

DISORDERS OF FETAL GROWTH

JOHN CATER
M.B., Ch.B., M.R.C.P.E., D.C.H.
Lecturer in Child Health
University of Aberdeen

Introduction

DEFINITION AND MEASUREMENT OF FETAL GROWTH

Growth is defined in the Concise Oxford Dictionary as an increase in size, height, or quantity. To the clinician, in broad terms, body growth is synonymous with increase in body mass and this is most easily assessed by serial measurement of weight. In normal intrauterine life, increasing weight can be assumed to represent the orderly process of growth. Abnormal weights at birth are clearly useful as indications of pathological conditions but a normal birth weight may be found in such abnormal growth situations as achondroplasia (25), hydrops or hydrocephalus, and the dangers of blindly accepting normal birth weight as being equated with normal growth are obvious.

Recent studies of cell numbers and size in babies of similar birth weight have further pin-pointed the difficulties of using weight as a criterion of growth. For example, two babies of identical weight may have very different cellular populations. The first may have a normal total number of cells but the individual cell is reduced in size whilst the other may have cells of normal size but reduced in number. From recent studies, it seems probable that reduction in cell size can be compensated for in ultimate post-natal growth but a deficiency in absolute numbers cannot (15).

Weight as a measure of growth takes no account of such dimensions as length or volume. It also ignores other processes, usually associated in the clinician's mind with growing, such as maturation of enzyme systems and neurological pathways. These systems, at least in the fetus, appear to be more closely related to gestational age than to weight. However, one must appreciate the advantages of weight as an index of growth in infancy and childhood: it is simple to measure, reliable, and easily reproducible.

NORMAL FETAL GROWTH

Growth as measured by an increase in weight, is made up of three fundamental processes. These are increase in cell number, increase in cell size, and the accumulation of non-living intercellular material. Superimposed upon this simple concept is the process of differentiation. Organ structure occurs as a result of tissue differentiation and the major part of this takes place in the embryonic period of intrauterine life. It is, however, during the fetal period that the greater part of the increase in size, as opposed to differentiation, occurs (11).

The mean daily intrauterine increase in body weight over the whole of pregnancy is approximately 12·5 g (31). The bulk of the increase in weight takes place in the second half of pregnancy. If one compares the mean weight of the fetus at 24 weeks with that of the fetus at term, the nett weight gain is approximately 2,300 g (14). A particularly rapid phase of growth takes place between the thirtieth and the thirty-sixth week, in singleton fetuses (17). After this stage it appears that the rate of growth (reflected by birth weights) is reduced.

Fat, for example, is only present in scanty amounts in the fetus before 20 weeks. At 28 weeks of gestation, it accounts for 3·5 per cent of body weight and at term a fetus weighing 3,500 g may consist of 16 per cent fat (31).

Growth in terms of absolute length occurs more slowly during the first 55 days (1 mm per day) than later (1·5 mm per day) (11). The mean crown–heel length of a newborn at term is approximately 50 cm (see chapter 1).

The head of the embryo, fetus and infant appears relatively large in comparison with the rest of the body. In infancy, the brain undergoes a linear increase in weight from birth until about 13 months of age and the final adult weight of 1,300 g is reached at about 6 years of age (31). As body structures continue growing there is a relative decrease in the size of the head compared with the rest of the body.

The measurement of growth is difficult enough in infancy but it is very much more difficult when considering the fetus. Due to the inaccessibility of the fetus, the clinician relies on simple abdominal palpation as his routine method of assessing growth which, in this context, is equated with an increase in size. The inappropriateness of such a criterion is clear when one remembers the course of events taking place from fertilization. Numerous tests for the estimation of fetal growth have been devised. Examples, such as ultrasonics, X-rays, and oestriol measurements are discussed at greater length in other parts of the book.

The state of growth of a particular newborn infant can be estimated by comparing certain measurements, e.g. weight, length, head circumference (occipito-frontal circumference) and other parameters, with standards derived from examination of large numbers of babies born at various known gestational ages. Although it is open to debate whether a pre-term infant can be considered representative of fetuses of equivalent gestation still in the uterus, such data in the form of distribution graphs, e.g. as percentile charts, are widely used as standards. Experience has shown that higher morbidity and mortality are found in babies with birth weights at the extremes of the frequency distribution (6). Babies whose birth weights fall below the tenth percentile or above the ninetieth percentile for gestation are commonly considered to be abnormally light or abnormally heavy respectively. Within these broad categories, however, a number of normal babies will be found and the use of more stringent criteria of abnormality has been suggested, for example, birth weights beyond the fifth and ninety-fifth percentiles, or birth weights more than 2 standard deviations below or above the means (two standard deviations below and above the mean correspond approximately to the third and ninety-seventh percentiles respectively). In terms of abnormal babies thus delineated, it seems that the use of the fifth and ninety-fifth percentiles as the basis of definition of normal growth is more meaningful. It must, however, be pointed out that this is a purely statistical approach to the growth of a fetus who is blissfully unaware of the delights of applied mathematics.

The clinical relevance of deviations from normal growth is evident in morbidity and mortality patterns. Fetuses which are disproportionately light for gestational age have an increased intrauterine mortality rate, particularly during labour as a result of asphyxia, and 'light-for-dates' infants tend to have a high incidence of hypoglycaemia, pulmonary haemorrhage, and pneumonia during the initial neonatal period.

'Heavy-for-dates' infants of longer gestations have an increased incidence of mechanical problems at delivery. An excess of infants of diabetic mothers is also found in this group. Broadly speaking, infants whose birth weights fall within the normal range tend to develop fewest problems for any given gestational age. Conversely, normal weight has its own distinctive morbidity pattern and infants of normal birth weight have an increasing likelihood of developing hyaline membrane disease with decreasing gestational age.

Similar graphs to those for weight have been constructed for other anthropometric measurements of the newborn infant in an attempt to delineate more clearly the pattern of fetal growth. Occipito-frontal circumference, crown-rump and crown-heel length, skinfold thickness and necropsy organ weight have been utilized. The relevance of these various parameters will be discussed below when describing the various charts used in delineating babies with disordered fetal growth (see Appendix 1).

FACTORS INFLUENCING FETAL GROWTH

A number of factors are known to influence the rate of fetal growth as reflected in variations of weight at birth. It is clearly preferable to use weight for gestational age charts that take at least some of these factors into account. A baby with a perfectly normal rate of growth may be recorded as having a birth weight below the tenth percentile because of failure of the clinician to appreciate the significance of pregnancy number and the sex of the infant on birth weight.

SEX

The difference in birth weight between males and females only becomes apparent after about the thirty-fourth week of gestation.

Males have a slightly greater weight gain from this stage onwards and by about 38 weeks weigh an average of 150 g more than females (30). The male at each gestational age has a greater crown-heel length, greater occipito-frontal circumference, and thinner skinfold measurements than the female (9).

MATERNAL PHYSIQUE

Maternal physical characteristics have a profound effect on the rate of fetal growth. When comparing, for example, the extremes of maternal physique, tall, heavy mothers (170 cm, 75 kilograms) with short, light mothers (150 cm, 40 kilograms), the average birth weight at term may be nearly 750 g greater in the infant of the former (30). Thomson, Billewicz, and Hytten (30) have published a table enabling correction of the birth weight to be made according to maternal height and weight at mid-pregnancy. Such a correction should be carried out before applying sex and pregnancy number adjustments to the birth weight.

PREGNANCY NUMBER

Birth weights in second and subsequent pregnancies, from about the thirty-second week onwards, are about 100 g heavier than in first pregnancies. The greater rate of fetal growth is thought to be due to the increase in vascularity of the multiparous uterus (30).

CIGARETTE SMOKING

This has a number of biological effects in the human; in relation to fetal growth, it has been shown to cause a reduction in the birth weight irrespective of the length of gestation (29).

MATERNAL NUTRITION

It is somewhat surprising to find that maternal nutritional deprivation must be very severe before birth weight is affected. Studies carried out following a period of severe war-time starvation in Holland (from September 1944 to May 1945) showed a greatly increased rate of amenorrhoea (50 per cent) with a diminished rate of conception (about one-third) during the period of famine. It was also shown that the average birth weight was only significantly reduced (240 g) if the mother was subjected to famine conditions during the last three to four and a half months of the pregnancy. Only the short, clearly-defined period (7 months) of severe nutritional deprivation in a previously well-nourished population made it possible to demonstrate the effects of starvation in this way (28).

RACE AND SOCIAL CLASS

It is well known that variations in average birth weight occur between different ethnic groups, irrespective of environment, and also between different socio-economic groups in a homogeneous population. Unfortunately, it is impossible to disentangle the effects of genetic factors from those of nutritional, socio-economic, and other environmental circumstances. There is a good deal of evidence, however, which shows that women born, reared, and reproducing in a good environment have a higher degree of reproductive efficiency which is undoubtedly associated with their better health and physique. Nevertheless, certain limits are set by genetic potential, for example, maternal height, to which birth weight is correlated.

Disordered fetal growth

TERMINOLOGY

With the decline in maternal mortality it was inevitable that attention would be directed towards the reduction of the perinatal death rate, which was highest amongst babies whose weights were 2,500 g or less.

The excessive mortality rate of the premature infant drew particular attention to this group, but the heterogeneous nature and expression of the disorders of growth contained within such a definition (birth weight of 2,500 g or less) have been increasingly appreciated. A brief review of the nomenclature is given in an attempt not only to explain the meaning of the various terms but also to show the clinical situation that the authors were describing.

REVIEW OF NOMENCLATURE

Prematurity. Though it has long been recognized that fetuses have different rates of intrauterine growth, it was convenient to have an international standard for comparative purposes. In the framing of the original definition, it was appreciated that such a term would not be necessarily relevant for every country. Prematurity was defined as a birth weight of 2,500 g or less. In the absence of a recorded birth weight, an infant of less than 37 weeks of gestation was defined as premature (33).

The results of the perinatal mortality survey showed that one-third of babies who weighed 2,500 g or less (i.e. 'premature by weight') were delivered after 38 weeks. Such infants were clearly not premature by date. Many terms have been coined which attempt to describe the problem of a variable rate of fetal growth. As yet, none is biologically precise and phonetically pleasing.

Dysmaturity. Sjostedt, Engelson, and Rooth (27) defined dysmaturity based on Clifford's placental dysfunction syndrome as a clinical syndrome which could occur at any gestational age, the clinical manifestations being grouped in three stages of severity.

1. The skin shows evidence of peeling and cracking or is of a parchment-like quality and the limbs are thin.
2. The skin changes are present to a greater degree than in stage 1. Though not in their original definition, they found as a result of their study that green staining had occurred in the nails, skin, or umbilicus, due to the presence of meconium in the amniotic fluid.
3. The skin peels off in large amounts and yellow staining of the skin, nails, and umbilical cord occurs. The infant shows marked thinning of the limbs and trunk (27).

Post-Maturity. It is said that all good things come to an end and this seems certainly true of the benevolent uterus. It has been customary to define post-maturity in terms of weeks of gestation and this proves extremely useful in clinical practice. At present the patho-physiological mechanisms of post-maturity are not understood. From studies of newborn birth weights there appears to be a reduction in the rate of weight gain after about the thirty-sixth week of gestation (17). The clinical manifestations of the post-mature newborn are well known, e.g. the dry, cracking, and peeling skin with loss of subcutaneous tissue.

Chronic fetal distress. Gruenwald introduced the term 'chronic fetal distress' to describe the intrauterine situation which results in an infant displaying the following features:

1. A birth weight below minus two standard deviations (corresponding to approximately the third percentile).
2. A reduction in body length and clinical evidence of malnutrition (loose skin and markedly diminished subcutaneous tissue).

He assumed that a birth weight below two standard deviations 'was an indication of retardation of growth' and that the associated finding of a reduction in body length for gestation was the result of a 'lengthy period of intrauterine deprivation'. Sub-acute fetal distress, which only rarely occurs in its classical form and is envisaged as lasting for a few days, manifests itself by a reduction in subcutaneous tissue, i.e. malnutrition. Body length is not significantly reduced giving the infant a long, thin appearance (10).

Fetal malnutrition. Scott and Usher used the term 'fetal malnutrition' to describe the features of the infant who is underweight for his age and/or shows clinical signs of soft tissue wasting (loose subcutaneous tissue and decreased muscle mass) (24).

Small-for-dates. The term originally embraced the same concept as Gruenwald's 'chronic fetal distress', namely, abnormally low birth weight and a reduction in body length. It is the term most widely used to describe babies who are growth retarded and has variously been defined as a birth weight below the tenth or fifth percentiles or below minus two standard deviations for gestational age.

When describing disorders of fetal growth and using weight for gestational age charts as the criterion, terminology relating to weight, i.e. light and heavy, is to be preferred to terms such as 'small' and 'large' which describe size. The term 'light-for-dates' should therefore be used in preference to the term 'small-for-dates' (20).

Dystrophic. This term is little used in the U.K. but is in frequent use in continental Europe. It merely implies defective or faulty nutrition of the fetus (32).

Small for gestational age, etc. (Denver classification). Battaglia and Lubchenco have recently introduced a new terminology based on the original Denver weight for gestational age chart. Babies are described as 'large for gestational age' (above the ninetieth percentile); 'appropriate for gestational age' (tenth to ninetieth percentiles); and 'small for gestational age' (below tenth percentile). By the additional use of pre-term, term, and post-term, newborn infants can be sub-divided into 9 separate groups, e.g. pre-term, small for gestational age (3).

RECENTLY PROPOSED CLASSIFICATION

Attempts have been made to clarify the terminology. At present 'low birth weight' is an internationally-accepted definition. A document proposing suggestions of definitions (Pre-term, Post-term and Term) was circulated at the Second European Congress of Perinatal Medicine in London, 1970 (34).

Low birth weight. Low birth weight is defined as a birth weight of 2,500 g or less, irrespective of the length of gestation. (World Health Organisation, 1961.)

Pre-term. Pre-term refers to a birth which occurs before 37 completed weeks of gestation (i.e. 259 days), irrespective of the birth weight.

Term. 37–41 weeks (259–93 days).

Post-term. 42 weeks or more (294 days) (34).

Light for dates. The light-for-dates baby is most commonly defined as a baby with a birth weight below the tenth percentile for a given gestational age (sometimes the fifth percentile or minus two standard deviations is used).

Heavy for dates. This term is commonly used when the birth weight is above the ninetieth percentile for gestational age.

Clinical relevance of disordered fetal growth

Deviations from normal fetal growth may result from genetic or environmental factors, or from a combination of both. Abnormality may be manifested in terms of reduced fetal growth, normal overall growth with selective reduction or excess of fetal growth. An attempt has been made in the following section to highlight the importance of the various types of abnormal and normal fetal growth.

LIGHT FOR DATES

Prompt diagnosis of the light-for-dates infant is of immense importance since hypoglycaemia, requiring prompt and energetic treatment, cerebral birth injury, with or without asphyxia, and intrapartum or neonatal pneumonia are all commoner in poorly-grown babies. Light-for-dates infants occur under the following circumstances:

Unknown aetiology. This comprises the vast majority of light-for-dates infants. Although a specific aetiology cannot be demonstrated, factors may be present in the mother, the pregnancy, the placenta or the umbilical cord which are often found in association with fetal growth retardation.

Reduction of fetal growth in association with congenital abnormalities. An increase in the incidence of congenital abnormalities is said to occur with a decrease in weight for gestation (7). Experiments on animals have shown that malformed embryos are smaller than their normal litter mates. At present, the mechanism responsible for the depression of the birth weight in such circumstances is poorly understood.

Evidence is available to show that reduction of fetal growth occurs in Trisomy 18 (25) and the 'cri du chat' syndrome. In a high proportion of fetuses with these two conditions, birth weights are below the tenth percentile for gestation. Abnormality of the sex chromosomes as in Turner's syndrome may result in considerable reduction in fetal growth (23). Infants with other chromosomal abnormalities, as in Down's syndrome, have a lower than expected birth weight when compared with the normal, though the reduction in birth weight is not normally in the pathological range. The rate of intrauterine growth in Trisomy 13–15 is reduced as reflected by a lower birth weight but to a lesser extent than in Trisomy 18 (23).

Infections. A number of intrauterine infections are associated with low birth weight, for example, toxoplasmosis, herpes simplex, syphilis, rubella, cytomegalovirus disease. Rubella has been clearly shown to cause reduction in the rate of fetal growth with a resultant light-for-dates infant. The virus may have the following effects upon the conceptus, inhibition of cell division (22), an increase in 'chromosomal breaks' (4) and an obliterative angiopathy affecting capillaries and other small blood vessels (8). The clinical manifestations of rubella virus infection depend entirely on the timing of the viral insult during pregnancy.

Placental causes (excluding post-maturity). Early workers who studied the subject of growth retardation assumed that placental insufficiency was responsible for the failure of certain fetuses to maintain normal growth. However, the search for constant, placental pathology in association with fetal growth retardation has proved most unrewarding. The rare pathological situation of parabiosis (circulatory shunting between monozygotic twin placenta) may result in the donor twin being much lighter than the recipient (18).

Severe pre-eclamptic toxaemia. Of all the grades of pre-eclampsia, only the most severe causes a reduction in birth weight. In babies delivered before term of mothers with severe P.E.T., most of the birth weights were below average. Such an effect on the birth weight was not obvious after term (1).

Small normal. When employing such an arbitrary criterion of abnormal growth as a percentile weight curve, it is inevitable that the abnormal group will include some babies who are small but normal.

Miscellaneous. Impairment in the rate of fetal growth has been described in a number of different syndromes. There are various types of low birth weight dwarfs such as Silver's syndrome (26) and the birdhead dwarfs of Seckel (12) which fall into the light-for-date category but these are very rare.

NORMAL WEIGHT FOR DATES

Pre-term infant. Survival of the infant is unusual if birth occurs at less than 28 weeks of gestation. From the practical point of view the problems presented depend upon the degree of 'premature expulsion' from the uterus. The physical characteristics of the newborn infant delivered at various gestational ages are described in the work of Farr and Mitchell (see Appendix 1). The incomplete maturation of certain functions results in the well-known problems of the pre-term infant, the most important of these clinically being:

1. The tendency to oedema and acidaemia.
2. Inability to maintain body temperature.
3. Development of respiratory distress.
4. Development of hyaline membrane syndrome.
5. Neonatal jaundice.
6. Susceptibility to infection.
7. Incomplete maturation of the nervous system with resultant disadvantages, e.g. absence of sucking reflex etc.

HEAVY FOR DATES

Fetuses with excessive birth weights are either pathological or represent the upper limits of biological variation. Heavy-for-dates infants are arbitrarily defined as those with birth weights above the ninetieth percentile. At least two distinct groups have been recognized in this weight range.

1. *Infants of diabetic mothers.* The classical appearance of a large plethoric infant is quite unmistakable. The excessive weight is not due to oedema (which may be present as part of the syndrome of immaturity), but to the increased deposition of fats (21). These fetuses show an increased body weight and crown–heel length (19) for gestation and growth rate in excess of normal. The surfeit of intrauterine nutrition is certainly not advantageous to the fetus.

On the one hand these infants suffer from the problems of shortened gestation such as hyaline membrane disease and increased neonatal jaundice, and on the other hand they suffer from profound disturbances of carbohydrate metabolism which may render them hypoglycaemic. Obviously their management by the neonatal paediatrician must take these factors into account and include:

a. Incubator care for the control of temperature and adequate observation.

b. Attention to the umbilical cord which is often excessively thick and requires care at ligature.

c. Prevention of hypoglycaemia.

2. *Transposition of the great vessels of the heart.* It has been noted that babies born with this abnormality have an increased rate of fetal growth as reflected by their birth weight. The biological mechanism of this is unknown, but it is not due to the presence of cardiac failure or oedema at birth. It has been recorded that transposition occurs more commonly in males and there may be a higher incidence of a family history of diabetes (16). It is important to recognize infants with transposition since the life-saving Rashkind procedure is now available in the newborn period.

OTHER RELEVANT GROUPS

Post-mature infant. The special clinical problem of post-mature (294 days) babies appears to be the increased mortality during labour. This was shown to be particularly so in first pregnancies. The risk diminished with increasing parity but even when considering the post-mature infant of the grand multipara it was found to have a 17 per cent increase in mortality rate when compared with a similar multiparous delivery at term (5).

Baird and Thomson (2) considered asphyxia and mechanical stress to be the main cause of perinatal mortality after term and pointed out that such deaths occurred with little or no warning and the most vulnerable group was the elderly primigravida. The underlying mechanisms suspected were:

a. Defective oxygenation of fetal blood after term.
b. Heavy fetus resulting in disproportion during labour.
c. Rigidity of cervix and uteric dysfunction in the elderly primigravida.
d. 'Placental insufficiency' in 'babies who are seriously under weight after term'.

Multiple pregnancy. The birth weight, body length, and occipito-frontal circumference of twins up to the thirty-fifth week are comparable to those of singletons. However, after the thirty-fifth week the products of multiple pregnancies show a significant reduction in these parameters when compared with single births (13). The aetiology of marked dissimilarity in the birth weights between monozygotic twins has already been discussed under placental pathology.

In conclusion, it can be said that the mechanisms responsible for regulation of fetal growth are not clearly understood. At present we are only beginning to appreciate the variety of expressions of abnormal growth in the newborn infant and it may be many years before the long-term significance of disturbances of fetal growth is fully evaluated.

References

1. BAIRD, D., THOMSON, A. M., and BILLEWICZ, W. Z. (1957). 'Birth-weights and placental weights in pre-eclampsia', *J. Obstet. Gynaec. Br. Commonw.*, **64**, 370.
2. —— —— (1969). 'Reduction of perinatal mortality by improving standards of obstetric care', *Perinatal Problems* (Edinburgh and London: E. and S. Livingstone).
3. BATTAGLIA, F. C., and LUBCHENCO, L. O. (1967). 'A practical classification of newborn infants by weight and gestational age', *J. Pediat.*, **71**, 159.
4. BOUE, A., and BOUE, J. G. (1969). 'Effects of rubella virus infection on the division of human cells', *Am. J. Dis. Child.* **118,** 45.
5. BUTLER, N. R., and BONHAM, D. G. (1963). *Perinatal Mortality* (Edinburgh and London: E. and S. Livingstone).
6. —— (1965). 'Perinatal death', *Clins. Devl. Med.*, **19**, 74.
7. DRILLEN, C. M. (1970). 'The small-for-date infant: etiology and prognosis', *Pediat. Clins. N. Am.*, **17**, 9.

8. DRISCOLL, S. G. (1969). 'Histopathology of gestational rubella', *Am. J. Dis. Child.*, **118**, 49.
9. GAMPEL, B. (1965). 'The relation of skinfold thickness in the neonate to sex, length of gestation, size at birth and maternal skinfold', *Hum. Biol.*, **37**, 29.
10. GRUENWALD, P. (1963). 'Chronic fetal distress and placental insufficiency', *Biologia Neonat.*, **5**, 215.
11. HAMILTON, W. J., BOYD, J. D., and MOSSMAN, H. W. (1945). 'Growth of the embryo: development of external form: estimation of the embryonic and fetal age', *Human Embryology* (Cambridge: Heffer).
12. HARPER, R. G., ORTI, E., and BAKER, R. K. (1967). 'Bird-headed dwarfs (Seckel's syndrome). A familial pattern of developmental, dental, skeletal and central nervous system anomalies', *J. Pediat.*, **70**, 799.
13. LUBCHENCO, L. O., HANSMAN, C., and BACKSTROM, L. (1968). *Aspects of Prematurity and Dysmaturity* (N. V. Leiden: H. E. Stenfert Kroesse).
14. —— ——, DRESSLER, M., and BOYD, E. (1963). 'Intrauterine growth as estimated from liveborn birthweight at 24–42 weeks of gestation', *Pediatrics*, **32**, 793.
15. MEDOVY, H. (1967). 'New parameters in neonatal growth-cell number and cell size', *J. Pediat.*, **71**, 459.
16. MEHRIZI, A., and DRASH, A. (1961). 'Birth weight of infants with cyanotic and acyanotic congenital malformations of the heart', *J. Pediat.*, **59**, 715.
17. McKEOWN, T., and RECORD, R. G. (1952). 'Observations on fetal growth in multiple pregnancy in man', *J. Endocr.*, **8**, 386.
18. NAEYE, R. L. (1963). 'Human intrauterine parabiotic syndrome and its complications', *New Engl. J. Med.*, **268**, 804.
19. —— (1965). 'Infants of diabetic mothers: a quantitative morphologic study', *Pediatrics*, **35**, 980.
20. NELIGAN, G. A. (1967). 'The clinical effects of being "light-for-dates" ', *Proc. R. Soc. Med.*, **60**, 881.
21. OSLER, M. (1960). 'Body fat of newborn infants of diabetic mothers', *Acta Endocr.*, **34**, 277.
22. PLOTKIN, S. A., BOUE, A., and BOUE, J. G. (1965). 'The in vitro growth of rubella virus in human embryo cells', *Amer. J. Epidem.*, **81**, 71.
23. REISMAN, L. E. (1970). 'Chromosome abnormalities and intrauterine growth retardation', *Pediat. Clins. N. Am.*, **17**, 101.
24. SCOTT, K. E., and USHER, R. (1966). 'Fetal malnutrition: its incidence, causes and effects', *Am. J. Obstet. Gynec.*, **94**, 951.
25. SCHUTT, W. H. (1965). 'Fetal factor in intrauterine growth retardation', *Clins. Devl. Med.*, **91**, 1.
26. SILVER, H. K. (1964). 'Assymetry, short stature and variations in sexual development', *Am. J. Dis. Child.*, **107**, 495.
27. SJOSTED, S., ENGELSON, G., and ROOTH, G. (1958). 'Dysmaturity', *Archs. Dis. Childh.*, **33**, 123.
28. SMITH, C. A. (1947). 'Effects of maternal undernutrition upon the newborn in Holland', *J. Pediat.*, **30**, 229.

29. TERRIS, M., and GOLD, E. M. (1969). 'An epidemiological study of prematurity. Relation to smoking, heart volume, employment and physique', *Am.J. Obstet. Gynec.*, **103**, 358.
30. THOMPSON, A. M., BILLEWICZ, W. Z., and HYTTEN, E. E. (1968). *J. Obstet. Gynaec. Br. Commonw.*, **75**, 903.
31. WIDDOWSON, E. M. (1970). 'Harmony of growth', *Lancet*, 901.
32. Dorland's Illustrated Medical Dictionary (1965). Twenty-fourth edition (Philadelphia and London: W. B. Saunders & Co.).
33. Manual of the International Statistical Classification of Diseases, Injuries, and Causes of Death. *Bull. Wld. Hlth. Org.*, Supp. 1, **1**, 212.
34. Suggestions of a Working Party of the Second European Congress of Perinatal Medicine (1970). 'Nomenclature of birthweight and gestational age', *Devl. Med. Child Neurol.*, **12**, 384.

Guides to further reading

'The small-for-date infant', ed. Andrews, B.F. (1970), *Pediat. Clins. N. Am.*, **17**, No. 1 (Philadelphia: W. B. Saunders and Co.).

LUBCHENCO, L. O., HANSMAN, C., and BACKSTROM, L. (1968). 'Factors affecting fetal growth', *Aspects of Prematurity and Dysmaturity*, Nutricia Symposium, eds. Jonxis, Visser, and Troelstra.

MEDOVY, H. (1967). 'New parameters in neonatal growth-cell number and size', *J. Pediat.*, **71**, 459.

SILVERMAN, W. A., and SINCLAIR, J. C. (1966). 'Infants of low birthweight', *New Engl. J. Med.*, **274**, 448.

SINCLAIR, J. C., and COLDIRON, J. S. (1969). 'Low birthweight and post-natal physical development', *Devl. Med. Child Neurol.*, **11**, 314.

CHAPTER 6

BLOOD GROUP ISO-IMMUNIZATION

Introduction

Blood group iso-immunization *has occurred when the fetal plasma contains maternal antibodies to fetal red cell antigens*. The iso-haemagglutinins (the normal blood group antibodies) are predominantly IgM and do not cross the placental barrier (see chapter 1), but immune antibodies, formed in the mother as a result of contact with antigens not present in her, are IgG and therefore transported through the placenta. Contact with a 'foreign' blood group antigen may occur by transplacental transfusion during pregnancy or treatment with unsuitable donor blood. A few vaccines, e.g. some diphtheria toxoids and influenza vaccines, contain traces of material from hog stomach or chick embryo which have been shown to stimulate the formation of immune antibodies in the recipient. Immune (IgG) antibodies crossing the placenta react with their antigens on the surface of the red cell. This reaction alters the surface structure of the red cell in such a way that they are removed from the circulation by the reticulo-endothelial system and broken down.

BLOOD GROUPS INVOLVED: THEIR INCIDENCE AND SCREENING

The Rhesus (Rh) antibodies are clinically most important

because of the severity of the haemolytic process and the high mortality rate. The Rhesus blood group system comprises several antigens of which D is that most commonly encountered in the clinical situation. These Rh antibodies complicate a maximum of 1 in 150–200 pregnancies. The incidence of immune ABO antibodies in pregnancy is 1 in 150 but the haemolytic disease caused is often very mild and such a figure represents the minimum incidence. Other blood group systems show a lower incidence and vary greatly in the severity of haemolysis associated.

TABLE 6.1.

System	*Haemolytic disease*	*Comment*	*Antibody occurrence without transfusion or pregnancy*
ABO	Yes	Mild form common	Regular
Rhesus	Yes	Often severe	Extremely rare
Kell	Yes	Rare	?
MNS	Yes	Very rare	Rare
P	No		Occasional
Lutheran	No		Extremely rare
Others	Very rare		

When pregnancy is diagnosed the blood groups of both parents should be ascertained and the mother's blood screened for the presence of abnormal antibodies. Antibodies are detected by an antiglobulin (Coomb's) test using cells from an individual having all the antigens that may be involved in iso-immunization. If antibodies are present they may be identified by agglutination tests against a panel of red cells each having a different antigen. The sensitivity of such methods is enhanced by the pre-treatment of the panel cells with enzymes such as ficin, bromelin, and papain. When an antibody is identified its titre is assayed and the assay repeated at intervals during the pregnancy. In the case of a Rh negative mother with Rh antibodies the genotype of the father should be found so as to assess the chance of a fetus being Rh positive, and the associated probability of a rise in antibody titre. The possibility of the presence of abnormal antibodies may be indicated by questions concerning previous blood transfusions and the incidence of neonatal jaundice in previous children.

DETECTION OF FETAL CELLS IN MATERNAL CIRCULATION

The extent of a leak of fetal blood into the mother's circulation is usually measured by the acid elution (Kleihauer) technique. The principle on which this method is based is that acid phosphate solutions will elute the adult haemoglobin (HbA) from adult cells but will not elute the fetal haemoglobin (HbF) from fetal cells. After suitable staining the fetal cells containing HbF and the adult 'ghost' red cells may be counted. If many fetal cells are present the volume of the leak may be estimated from counting the fetal and adult cells on the slide. If few fetal cells, then 50 low power fields are scanned and HbF cells counted. This is equivalent, approximately, to viewing 50,000 red cells and the ratio may thus be calculated.

FREQUENCY AND SIGNIFICANCE OF FETAL LEAKS

Just after delivery fetal cells may be detected in the blood of 50–60 per cent of mothers. The volume of blood transfused varies greatly. Commonly it is in the range of 0·04 to 4·0 ml but figures of more than 100 ml have been reported. Large transfusions of fetal blood are usually associated with pregnancies complicated by pre-eclampsia, accidental haemorrhage and uterine manipulation, as at lower segment caesarean section or manual removal of the placenta. Fetal leaks into the maternal circulation also occur earlier in pregnancy especially in the third trimester and have also been shown to occur during abortion, particularly surgical termination.

Rh positive fetal cells may remain in the circulation of a Rh negative mother for many weeks when mother and fetus are ABO compatible. However, when they are ABO incompatible fetal cells are found less often at delivery and remain in the circulation for a much shorter time. The removal of ABO incompatible cells depends on whether the fetus has developed the A or B antigens and also on the maternal α and β isohaemagglutinin titre. It is found that the incidence of maternal anti-D antibody formation is less when the fetus and mother are ABO incompatible. For first affected pregnancies the incidence of Rh antibodies where there is ABO incompatibility is 1 per cent as opposed to 8·5 per cent when there is ABO compatibility. The titre of anti-D formed seems to correlate well with the amount of blood transfused from the fetus into the mother. However, the amount of antibody formed at primary immunization does not correlate with that formed during subsequent affected pregnancies. Antibody formed early in a second pregnancy indicates a previous primary response even though in a few cases no fetal cells will have been detected after the first pregnancy. This presents a difficulty as regards the indications for anti-D treatment (see below).

A higher percentage (approximately twice) of women show an antibody response after the second pregnancy than after the first.

EFFECTS OF INCREASED HAEMOLYSIS

While the fetus is in utero, bilirubin is rapidly cleared via the placenta. Despite this, in a severely affected infant the cord blood levels of bilirubin may be elevated (above a maximum acceptable level of about 2·8 mgs per cent of total bilirubin). The conjugating enzymes necessary to convert the (unconjugated) bilirubin, produced from haemolysis (which is not very water soluble and is carried by albumin and β-lipoprotein), to the water soluble (conjugated) type excreted in the bile are considerably lower in the fetal liver than in the liver of an adult. Hence the rapid haemolysis causes its accumulation in the blood and it may pass through the blood-brain barrier with consequent damaging effects. In infants dying in this condition, unconjugated bilirubin is found in the basal ganglia where it causes yellow staining (hence the term kernicterus) and focal necrosis. After the first few days of post-natal life unconjugated bilirubin does not easily cross the blood-brain barrier. The danger of kernicterus is aggravated by the fact that fetal levels of protein and β-lipoprotein which hold unconjugated bilirubin in the circulation are low.

The extent of such haemolysis depends on the titre of antibodies produced in the maternal plasma and the length of time during which the fetus is exposed to them during gestation.

FACTORS AFFECTING THE PROBABILITY OF RH DISEASE IN THE INFANTS OF RHESUS NEGATIVE WOMEN

1. Previous transfusion of a Rh negative woman with Rh positive blood.
2. Increasing parity, as this increases the possibility of transplacental transfusion.
3. Pre-eclampsia or uterine manipulation during delivery is associated with increased volumes of fetal cells in the maternal circulation.
4. Paternal genotype. If the father is homozygous Rh positive then all his children will be Rh positive.
5. ABO group of the fetus. If the transfused cells are compatible they are not destroyed by maternal iso-haemagglutinins and have been shown to survive longer. This longer survival time gives a greater opportunity for stimulation of antibody formation.
6. Antibody formation in previous pregnancies. Immunological 'memory' facilitates the speed and titre of antibody formation on restimulation by the antigen.

ASSESSMENT OF MATERNAL ANTIBODIES

Maternal antibody titre is measured by an indirect antiglobulin (Coomb's) test. The purpose of this test is to find the titre of antibodies to Rh positive (usually D) cells. Maternal serum is mixed with Rh positive red cells so that any anti-Rh immune (IgG) antibody present will coat the cells. These coated cells are termed sensitized. The cells are washed to remove unattached antibody and mixed with serum containing antibodies to human IgG protein (viz. an antiglobulin serum). These antiglobulin antibodies (mostly IgM) complex with the IgG on the sensitized cells causing agglutination which is visible to the naked eye. Dilutions of maternal serum are made and the highest dilution to give agglutination is recorded; this dilution is termed the titre of the antibody. This test should be repeated at intervals to ascertain if there is a rise in the titre, which indicates an increased risk to the fetus.

In the first affected pregnancies, if the titre is less than 1 : 20 at 36 weeks the risk of fetal death is 0·3 per cent, but if greater than 1 : 20 at this time 16·5 per cent. As 50 per cent of affected infants are lost before 35 weeks, an indirect antiglobulin test should be performed at 12–14 weeks and if no antibodies are detected it should be repeated at 28 and 34 weeks. In any pregnancy a titre of greater than 1 : 20 is regarded as an indication for amniotic fluid examination after about 24 weeks. These figures refer to indirect antiglobulin tests by the tile technique; figures for the tube technique are higher.

It must be remembered that antibody titres alone are not a reliable guide to the severity of haemolytic disease. Recently, maternal serum antibody nitrogen has been used to assess the need for amniocentesis. The antibody nitrogen and the direct antiglobulin test titres correlate well in at least 95 per cent of cases. The advantage of antibody nitrogen is that it can be measured using an automated system. The method depends on measurement of haemoglobin released from Rh positive cells which remain unagglutinated after incubation with the test serum. The results are obtained by comparison of the tests with standards containing known amounts of anti-Rh antibody expressed as nitrogen. In first affected pregnancies, amniotic fluid examination is indicated if the antibody nitrogen is 1·5 μg/ml or more before the 34th week. In subsequent pregnancies a value of 0·5–1·0 μg/ml is probably sufficient indication.

Antibody quantitation of amniotic fluid may be of value in assessing the severity of fetal haemolysis.

ASSESSMENT OF THE SEVERITY OF FETAL HAEMOLYSIS

When the antiglobulin titre rises to 1 : 20 amniocentesis should be performed at 28–32 weeks and repeated at 2–3 week intervals as necessary. If there is a history of a previous affected infant requiring treatment, or still-birth or neonatal death due to haemolytic disease, amniocentesis should be considered at 24–30 weeks. Amniotic fluid samples are centrifuged at high speed to sediment debris and the supernatant fluid used to estimate the pigment level. Much of this pigment consists of compounds other than bilirubin and most methods measure some of these other compounds in addition to bilirubin. If the specimen cannot be assayed immediately it should be kept in the dark at 4°C. The optical density (O.D.) of amniotic fluid at 460 nm is due largely to bilirubin. The O.D. is not proportional to the bilirubin concentration, but by using a set of standards the concentration may be estimated. Liley measured the O.D. over the range 350–600 nm. Samples with no bilirubin show a fall in O.D. from 350–600 nm. The presence of bilirubin produces a hump at 460 nm. The height of this peak above the normal slope, in O.D. units is measured (Fig. 6.1.). Knox measured the ratio of O.D. at 490 nm to that at 520 nm on the grounds that above and below these wavelengths the O.D. is

FIG. 6.1. *Optical density of amniotic fluid from 350–630 nm.*

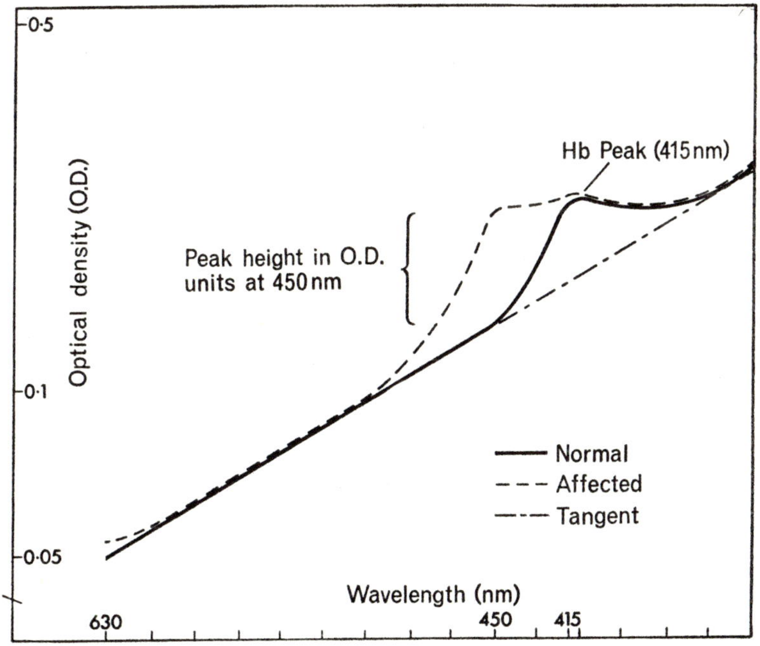

greatly affected by the presence of oxyHb. The results of such tests relate well to the survival of the affected fetus and have been claimed to give some prediction of the cord Hb at birth.

The amount of pigment in amniotic fluid tends to fall in parallel with the protein concentration as term is approached. Both the bilirubin and the protein have been measured to obtain a pigment : protein ratio in the belief that this may give a more accurate prediction.

Multiple examinations are required whichever method is used and the results may be plotted against the gestation time. Extrapolation of the line obtained indicates the prognosis and helps the obstetrician to decide the best time of delivery. Such tests have been found most accurate when the levels of pigment are very high or low. Because of variation in the middle range it is often difficult to find a line so as to predict when the fetus may be in danger.

Obstetric management

As indicated previously, measurement of the maternal antibody titres together with estimation of the bilirubinoid pigment in the liquor amnii, where indicated, guide the clinician in the obstetric management of the Rh-sensitized patient. Ideally he will allow the pregnancy to proceed and induce labour between 36 and 38 weeks, when the fetus is mature, and employ exchange transfusion as necessary. Good results are usually obtained if this line of management is adopted. However, if the severity of the haemolytic process warrants it, induction of labour may be indicated at 34 or 35 weeks or even earlier, followed by the birth of an affected immature infant, with a consequent decreased chance of survival. As over half the intrauterine deaths occur before 35 weeks, techniques have been devised to reduce the severity of the haemolytic process thus allowing the pregnancy to proceed longer.

INTRAUTERINE TRANSFUSION

Ideally an exchange transfusion in utero would be the solution to the problem of negotiating the knife edge between severity and immaturity. Rh negative blood, unaffected by the maternal antibodies would then replace the Rh positive blood of the fetus. This would reduce the haemolysis, increase the haemoglobin, and prevent hydropic changes. Attempts have been made to do this either by bringing out a loop of umbilical cord, or a fetal lower limb through a uterine incision. The umbilical cord, or in the second method, the femoral vein was catheterized. However, to carry out such a manoeuvre requires prolonged general anaesthesia, an abdominal incision, and replacement of the liquor, and has been followed by premature labour in most reported cases, although there is at least one successfully treated case using the lower limb.

Transfusion of the Rh negative blood into the fetus, without exchange, the intrauterine transfusion (I.U.T.), has now become widely accepted in the management of badly affected pregnancy. It is technically more feasible than the other methods mentioned above and it can be repeated during the pregnancy. Results are encouraging. The blood is injected into the peritoneal cavity of the fetus, and the red cells are absorbed into the fetal circulation via the sub-diaphragmatic lymphatics within 3–7 days.

The whole aim of the I.U.T. is to allow the pregnancy to proceed to 35 weeks when induction of labour is performed. It is performed to prevent intrauterine death, and must be carried out before the fetus is very severely affected.

The principal indications are:

1. History of fetal loss due to Rh haemolytic disease.
2. Increasing evidence of haemolysis from optical density measurements at 450 nm on liquor amnii.

Serial measurements are plotted on a prediction chart (Fig. 6.2) and, where the optical density differences increase into upper and upper middle zones, I.U.T. will be indicated. This decision depends on the stage of gestation and the steepness of the rise in relation to the normally decreasing levels, as pregnancy progresses.

The procedure commences with the intra-amniotic injection of a radio-opaque material, e.g. Urografin, or Myodil. This is

FIG. 6.2. *Amniotic fluid zones.*

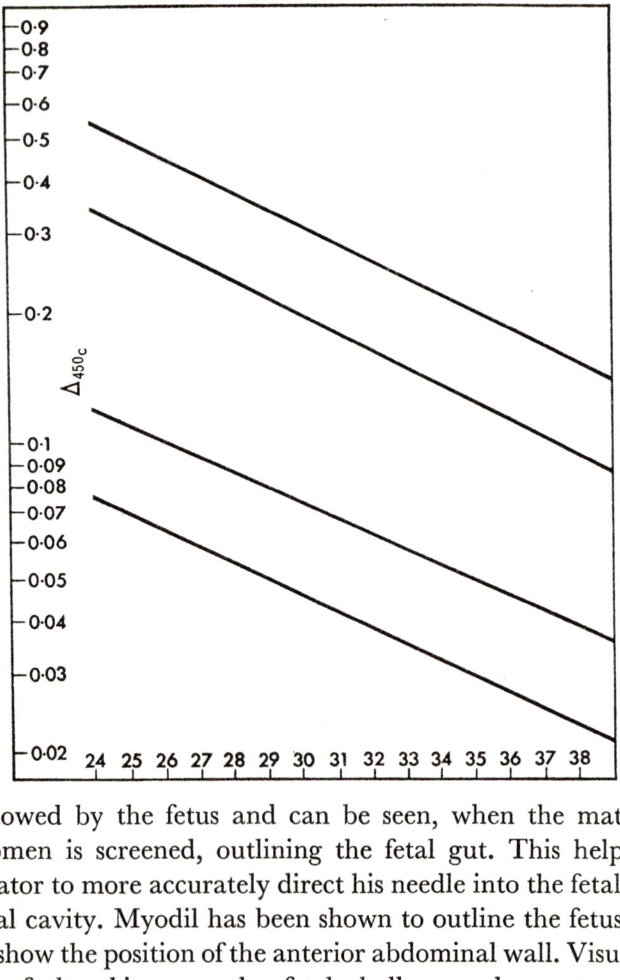

swallowed by the fetus and can be seen, when the maternal abdomen is screened, outlining the fetal gut. This helps the operator to more accurately direct his needle into the fetal peritoneal cavity. Myodil has been shown to outline the fetus also, and show the position of the anterior abdominal wall. Visualization of the skin over the fetal skull may demonstrate the presence of oedema in a hydropic baby.

The transfusion is carried out on the following day. A suitable premedication is given beforehand, and the patient is taken to the X-ray department, where complete asepsis must be observed. An image intensifier with television screen is essential, and markers are placed on the skin in relation to the position of the fetal gut.

Under local anaesthesia, a suitable needle, usually a 20 cm Touhy needle, is passed through the maternal anterior abdominal wall, the uterine wall, the fetal abdominal wall, and into the fetal peritoneal cavity. A small amount of radio-opaque dye is introduced to verify the correct positioning of the needle. Dye in the peritoneal cavity shows characteristic patterns of biconcave shadows between the loops of bowel and sub-diaphragmatic crescents. A plastic catheter 60–80 cm long is passed through the needle and the latter is withdrawn. Self-retaining catheters have been used where repeated transfusions are contemplated but leakage of blood into the amniotic cavity may occur.

Packed cells of fresh Rh negative blood of the same ABO group as the mother, concentrated to about 20 g haemoglobin per 100 ml blood, are injected slowly at a rate of 1–3 ml per minute. This is done manually using a syringe, or an automatic pump may be used. The volume of blood given depends on stage of gestation, and as the main concern is to provide red cells, the blood is 'packed'. The amount usually given is 70 ml per 1,000 g of fetal weight. The amount of transfused blood at 24, 28, and 32 weeks is thus in the region of 45, 75, and 120 ml respectively.

The procedure is repeated every 1 to 3 weeks until delivery is planned, in order that the adult blood given shall occupy 90–5 per cent of the total and the haemoglobin level of the fetus remains at a satisfactory level.

Vaginal delivery is usually allowed, unless there are obstetric indications for caesarean section.

Hazards. Radiation exposure to the fetus is kept to a minimum, but repeated transfusions are often necessary.

Maternal damage is rare, but accidental haemorrhage and bleeding from the uterus have been described. Injuries to the maternal bladder and bowel are rare.

The risk of trauma to the fetus by the needle is greater. Pleural cavity, liver, diaphragm, intestine, bladder, and skull may be damaged. Infection is always potentially dangerous, and routine antibiotic cover is advisable.

Intrauterine death has been hastened where the procedure has been carried out on hydropic infants. Presumably the increase in the circulation produced, worsens the already precarious cardiac state. Hydropic change can be detected radiologically and also by the presence of ascites, as evidenced by aspiration of the peritoneal contents before injecting the blood. About one-fifth of the cases go into premature labour. However, in many cases this has not prevented a favourable outcome.

Results. It is often difficult to assess results, and even more difficult to compare published series. 20–60 per cent survival rates have been claimed, and ideally these figures should represent a saving of infants who would otherwise have died. Results are much worse with hydropic infants, and also where the condition has been severe enough to warrant early intrauterine transfusions.

The technique should only be performed in Centres taking a special interest in, and with experience of, the problem.

THE PREVENTION OF RH ISO-IMMUNIZATION

Immunoglobulin containing a high titre of Rh antibodies (Anti-D), if given within 36 hours of delivery, will clear the fetal Rh positive cells that have leaked across into the maternal circulation. By this means, sensitization and subsequent production of Rh antibodies is prevented and a future pregnancy will be unaffected. This has proved a very successful procedure and is ineffective only where the leaks are very large. The amount administered to the mother is 200 μg which can clear leaks up to 30–40 ml of fetal blood. The presence and amount of the leaks can be assessed by the Kleihauer test, described above. The immunoglobulin is usually given after first deliveries in Rh negative women but when supplies are available there is good reason to administer it after subsequent deliveries, and also after abortion, particularly when performed therapeutically.

The preparations are commonly obtained by plasmaphoresis of Rh negative women who already have a high titre of Rh antibodies. Deliberate sensitization of males and post-menopausal women also provides a source. Clearly, as the whole problem is being slowly eradicated in the reproducing female population, these latter sources will become the main supply. Suitable commercial preparations are available.

Note. It is possible that soon the amount of antibody given will be reduced from 200 μg to 100 μg.

References and guides to further reading

'The antenatal diagnosis of rhesus incompatibility', *Perinatal Medicine* (1969). Ed. Huntingford, P. J., Huter, E. A., and Saling, E. (Stuttgart: Georg Thieme Verlag).

CLARKE, C. A. (1967). 'Prevention of Rh-haemolytic disease', *Br. Med. J.*, **4**, 7.

DACIE, J. V. (1967). 'Haemolytic disease of the newborn', *The Haemolytic Anaemias*, Part IV (London: Churchill).

FRASER, I. D. 'Uses of antibody nitrogen in assessment of Rhesus iso-immunization.' Personal communication.

FREDA, V. J. (1965). 'The Rh problem in obstetrics and a new concept in its management using amniocentesis and spectrophotometric scanning of amniotic fluid', *Am. J. Obstet. Gynec.*, **92**, 341.

KARNICKI, J. (1968). 'Results and hazards of prenatal transfusion', *J. Obstet. Gynaec. Br. Commonw.*, **75**, 1209.

LILEY, A. W. (1963). 'Errors in the assessment of haemolytic disease from amniotic fluid', *Am. J. Obstet. Gynec.*, **86**, 485.

—— (1965). 'The use of amniocentesis and fetal transfusion in erythroblastosis fetalis', *Pediatrics*, **35**, 836.

MORRIS, E. D., MURRAY, J., and RUTHVEN, C. R. J. (1967). 'Liquor bilirubin levels in normal pregnancy. A basis for accurate prediction of haemolytic disease', *Br. Med. J.*, **2**, 352.

SAVAGE, R. D., WALKER, W., FAIRWEATHER, D. V. I., and KNOX, E. G. (1966). 'Quantitative estimation of bilirubin in liquor amnii', *Lancet*, **2**, 816.

WOODROW, J. C., and DONOHOE, W. T. A. (1968). 'Rh-immunization by pregnancy. Results of a survey and their relevance to prophylactic therapy', *Br. Med. J.*, **4**, 139.

ZIPURSKY, A., POLLOCK, J., NEELANDS, P., CHOWN, B., and ISRAELS, L. G. (1963). 'The transplacental passage of fetal red blood cells and the pathogenesis of Rh immunization during pregnancy', *Lancet*, **2**, 489.

CHAPTER 7

DRUGS AND THE FETUS

Although a good deal is known of the effects of drugs on the human fetus and the volume of this knowledge increases almost daily, there remains a good deal of confusion in correlating what are often conflicting reports. Much work remains to be done and owing to the difficulties of such researches, many compounds remain untested with regards to their effects on the fetus. Consequently, many manufacturers simply state that their product should not be prescribed to pregnant women.

It came to be realized in 1961 that the sedative Thalidomide was a powerful teratogen and shortly thereafter the full enormity of the aftermath of its administration to pregnant women became apparent. This disastrous situation focused the attention of not only the medical world but also the general public on the possibility of a drug, which was regarded as safe, being of irreparable harm to the fetus. But there were positive sides too. It lent irresistible weight to the arguments for caution in allowing drugs on the market which had been insufficiently tested; for caution in prescribing for pregnant women; for a review of many of the drugs already given to pregnant women; and it stimulated much research into teratogenicity and congenital anomalies in general.

One of the great difficulties in assessing any therapeutic (or other) compound with regard to the possibility of harmful effects on the fetus is that experimental methods must of necessity be indirect.

Animal experiments are frequently employed, rodents being the most usual experimental animal. Such work yields valuable information but it is obvious that there are great interspecies differences and the results are not necessarily applicable to man. Moreover, interpretation of results is far from simple and the evaluation of the danger of teratogenicity of a compound is a complex matter.

Cytogenetic studies also yield highly significant information. Chromosome and chromatid breaks and other forms of gross disruption detectable by the microscope are produced by a number of compounds. It is possible to examine such effects in vitro, by tissue culture, using a large variety of cell lines including human and human fetal cells. In vivo experiments are possibly more valuable and again animals may be used, but it is also possible to examine in vivo effects in non-pregnant humans in many cases. Elaborate as these techniques are, they are relatively crude as far as the possibility of detecting genetic damage goes. Even when cytogenetic damage can be seen to be caused, this cannot be taken as proof of teratogenicity.

Revision of the legal position regarding the termination of pregnancy in the U.K. and some other countries has rendered available human material for study which was theretofore almost inaccessible. It is to be expected that from this source a great deal of new information regarding the effects of drugs on the fetus will be forthcoming.

Other sources of such information in humans are from sporadic reports, therapeutic accidents, and retrospective studies. Such material is usually inconclusive and very difficult to evaluate but can be useful in conjunction with results of other methods of study in building up as comprehensive a picture as possible. One danger, however, is that it is all too easy to build up an alarmist attitude (as it is possible to indicate almost anything by citing examples, and in this matter positive results remain in the medical and public mind longer than negative ones) and although it is impossible to be too careful in prescribing to women who are, or may be, pregnant it would be all too easy to condemn many of the most useful and effective drugs in the present therapeutic armamentarium.

In later pregnancy, the fear of teratogenicity becomes less but there is no cause for complacency. Most drugs have side effects, so why not on the fetus? This is apt to be overlooked because the fetus is not directly visible and cannot complain. Although the processes of organogenesis are completed with the end of the embryonic period of development, the fetus is still the site of very rapidly dividing cells and is thus presumably highly susceptible to many extraneous compounds in the same way as, for instance, the bone marrow is.

Study of the problem at this stage is scarcely less problematic than in the earlier stages but examination of aborted material, amniocentesis, (see chapter 4) and fetal blood sampling in labour (see chapter 2) are ways in which the fetus is becoming more accessible to the researcher and clinician. Radiological outlining and study of the fetus during intrauterine transfusion (see chapter 5) is yet another way in which the privacy of the fetus is being invaded. But these are all ways which can be adapted to the study of the effects of drugs.

In addition to all the necessary laboratory and clinical work, a strong case can be made for an organization for the central collection, sifting and correlation of data from all the various sources so that each drug may be evaluated on as much evidence as possible.

Even superficial acquaintance with the established facts of fetal physiology reveal that there are many vast differences when compared with that of the newborn or older individual. This is a fundamental which must be borne in mind when considering the effects of drugs upon the fetus. Definite facts regarding fetal pharmacology are scarce and difficult to come by, so that at the present state of knowledge, therapeutic recommendations can often only be made in the light of inference and surmise and consequently with great caution.

At the present time, therapeutic substances are seldom administered directly to the fetus although it is very likely that this will shortly change, radio-opaque substances and blood are already given in this way in the course of intrauterine transfusion. The main route of access of drugs to the fetus are via the placenta or the amniotic fluid.

The transfer of such substances across the placenta is thus an important consideration, but it is also necessary to consider transfer back to the maternal circulation of both the substance and its breakdown products. This is dependent on more than just placental 'permeability', but also presumably on other factors such as protein binding in mother and in fetus, renal function in the fetus, differential rates of metabolism in mother and fetus, placental function and probably many others.

Substances gaining access to the liquor amnii may reach the fetus directly through its permeable skin in early pregnancy or via its gastro-intestinal tract in later pregnancy. When there is an appreciable output of fetal urine into the liquor, the drug itself or its breakdown products may reach the liquor and be available for re-ingestion by the fetus.

One of the significant differences in pharmacology of the fetus is that enzymes active after birth often appear to be absent or inactive, and substances whose pharmacology in the adult is well known may not be metabolized in the same way.

Routes of excretion are also different. Excretion by the urine, as has been said, is not the same as after birth when urine is completely discarded; volatile substances cannot be excreted through the lungs, and the biliary and gastro-intestinal routes are not available. The main onus of excretion falls upon the placenta, whose pharmacological activities are obviously a crucial part of the problem.

Allowances must be made for the stage of gestation, as such things as renal function, placental function, absorption from swallowed liquor, permeability of the fetal skin, and the physico-chemical composition of the liquor all change as pregnancy proceeds.

The therapeutic situations which expose the fetus to the action of drugs and therapeutic regimens are considered here under four main headings:

1. *Drugs given directly to the fetus.* This has already been mentioned. Although instances are few at present, the possibility of direct access exists and is likely to prove irresistible, so that rapid developments in this sphere may be expected.
2. *Drugs given to the mother to secure a desired effect on the fetus.* These are also not numerous. Abortifacients are dealt with below. Antibiotics may be given to a mother who does not deliver her baby within an arbitrary interval of rupture of the membranes (often 24–48 hours) as a prophylactic measure against uterine infection and congenital pneumonia. Other examples such as administration of phenobarbitone when hyperbilirubinaemia is expected and prophylactic vitamin K can also be cited. Dietary restriction in mothers heterozygous for phenylketonuria has been advocated, the rationale being to prevent harmful exposure of the developing C.N.S. to the raised levels of phenylalanine found in such women.
3. *Drugs given to the mother for diagnostic or therapeutic reasons which may cross the placenta and affect the fetus.* These are obviously numerous and in the case of many drugs the effects, if any, on the fetus are simply not known. Even the ability of many therapeutic agents to cross the placenta is in many cases poorly documented.

   In instances where the fetus is delivered shortly after administration of the substance in question, as with the anaesthetics, more information on drug effect is available from monitoring before and during delivery, and resuscitation problems and general examination after delivery.

   Where sufficient information is not available, prescribing for a pregnant woman must always take into account possible effects on her unborn child. In some instances the position is unavoidable as may happen in women who suffer from conditions such as epilepsy.
4. *Drugs given to women who may be pregnant.* This is probably the most difficult group of all. Drug prescribing is now so commonplace that there can be few people who have escaped it altogether and some substances, e.g. codeine, salicylates, and purgatives, are available over the counter. The em-

bryonic period of development is a maximal risk time for malformation and it may be largely completed by the time pregnancy is suspected. Consequently, women may have prescribed for them, or may already be taking, drugs which might have been withheld were the medical attendant aware of the pregnancy.

Types of damage to the fetus

ABORTION

A baby born with a major malformation might be regarded as a reproductive near-miss and the high proportion of abnormal fetuses found amongst spontaneous abortions suggests that wider misses are dealt with in this way by nature.

Substances which produce abortions usually do so by differentially poisoning the mother and the fetus. If the process is insufficient to kill either, interference with the development of the fetus may result in abnormality. Ingested abortifacients range from potent cytotoxic agents such as the nitrogen mustards to poisons such as lead compounds. Quinine is also credited with the ability to produce abortion; and there are many others, claims for their efficacy stemming from fact or folk-lore, or both. It is important to remember that such compounds are usually dangerous poisons, and most act by this mechanism and not because they are specifically abortifacient.

TERATOGENICITY

Something has already been said about teratogenicity. The precise effect produced depends upon the teratogen reaching the conceptus, the concentration which it achieves there and the stage of development at which exposure occurs. It is likely that there are several mechanisms capable of producing such changes, and possible that different mechanisms may operate for the same teratogen at different developmental stages.

Vitamin deficiencies, local or general, may interfere with cell proliferation, and there is at least circumstantial evidence to suggest that some compounds (e.g. thalidomide, aminopterin) may produce their effects in this way. Ionizing radiations have varying effects on different cell populations but may produce hypertrophy, interruption of mitosis or cell death which may in turn lead to malformation (vide infra).

Lysergic acid diethylamide causes chromosomal breaks similar to those produced by X-rays. These have been observed in users and offspring of users, and increased abortion and malformation rates have been described in rats treated with this substance.

ADVERSE EFFECTS ON FUNCTION

In an anatomically normal fetus adverse effects on function constitute a type of effect frequently encountered and of practical importance to the obstetrician and paediatrician. Examples are the depression of respiratory function which may be produced by sedative and anaesthetic drugs given during labour, and the depression of coagulating mechanisms associated with anticonvulsant therapy to the mother. A more detailed account of such effects is given in the section below dealing with individual compounds.

RADIATIONS

The hazards of ionizing radiations to the fetus are now well documented. Deleterious effects range from gross damage with cell necrosis to the production of abnormalities which may not become manifest until well into post-natal life.

X-rays. The effects of X-rays on the developing organism have been extensively studied, and it seems that these are multiple and complicated. They do more than merely interrupt mitosis as evidenced by the fact that the adverse effects may be considerably delayed, in terms of cell generations, from the damaging exposure.

Atomic radiation. Analysis of results of human pregnancies exposed to atomic radiation, sufficient to produce clinical effects in the mother after the atomic bomb explosion in Nagasaki, showed a very much increased incidence of abortion, neonatal and infant deaths and abnormal children (mainly C.N.S. abnormality). The overall catastrophe rate in mothers exposed to radiation, but not showing major signs, was only slightly raised compared with the control group.

Ultrasonics. Ultrasonic radiations are coming to be increasingly used in pregnancy. No deleterious effects on the fetus have been recorded, and it is claimed that such procedures are safe and may in some clinical situations spare the fetus the hazards of X-rays. There have been a few recent hints, based on animal experiments, that ultrasonic radiations of higher energy than those used diagnostically may produce harmful effects. It is perhaps appropriate to bear in mind that X-radiation had been in use for years before some of its destructive effects were fully appreciated.

VACCINES

Much that applies to drugs in respect of the difficulty of establishing definite facts concerning safety or otherwise also applies to vaccines. Whereas drugs are most often used therapeutically, vaccines are prophylactic. Because of this, the timing of administration can often be chosen to avoid giving vaccines to pregnant women. However, in the face of an epidemic, administration may have to be undertaken even if the risks are great, as may happen, for example, with smallpox. In considering individual vaccines, it seems relevant to divide these into live and killed vaccines.

Live vaccines. Vaccination against smallpox should be avoided in pregnant women and their close family (see chapter 8 on maternal smallpox and vaccinia).

Rubella: this vaccine should not be given to pregnant women. The 'wild' virus carries such a high risk of producing embryopathy (see chapter 8) that it is prudent not to expose pregnant women to the 'tame' virus. In any case, there are no indications to give the vaccine to women who are already pregnant.

Yellow fever: this vaccine is strongly contra-indicated during pregnancy.

Measles: this vaccine, like that of rubella, probably need never be used during pregnancy.

Poliomyelitis: like other like vaccines, viraemia occurs after live polio vaccine and on general principles this should be avoided during pregnancy. It is likely that some pregnant women do come into contact with the virus with recently 'vaccinated' people. Moreover, as the live vaccine offers the only prospect of containing an on-going epidemic, circumstances may occur under which it may have to be given.

When a live vaccine such as vaccinia or rubella has to be administered to a woman of reproductive age, it is a sensible precaution to first enquire about the possibility of early pregnancy and to advise that appropriate steps in avoiding pregnancy be taken over the ensuing three months.

Killed vaccines. The majority of these are probably safe during pregnancy.

Diphtheria and Pertussis are unlikely to be required during pregnancy.

Tetanus may have to be given but often as a 'booster' to an already immunized adult.

Typhoid (T.A.B.), Cholera, and Typhus immunizations may be required in connection with travel to endemic areas or in epidemic times. These may produce a febrile reaction shortly after administration but side effects are mainly local and probably carry little or no risk to the fetus.

Relevant information on individual drugs

In the following section, a number of drugs are dealt with individually with respect to the effects on the fetus. The list is, naturally, very incomplete and the selection has been made from a clinical viewpoint. The fetus will be exposed to many of the drugs mentioned more by accident than design, and it can be seen from this how deficient the knowledge is concerning some of these.

ANAESTHETICS

Volatile anaesthetics Local anaesthetics Basal anaesthetics Muscle relaxants Atropine

ANTIBIOTICS

Penicillins Tetracyclines Streptomycin Chloramphenicol

CHEMOTHERAPEUTIC AGENTS

Sulphonamides Trimethoprim Nalidixic acid Nitrofurantoin

ANTICOAGULANTS

Heparin Coumarol derivatives

ANTICONVULSANTS

Barbiturates Phenytoin Primidone Ethosuximide

ANTIHISTAMINES

Chlorpheniramine Promethazine

ANTIHYPERTENSIVES

Guanethidine Methyldopa Reserpine

DIURETICS

Frusemide Chlorthiazide

HORMONES AND DRUGS ACTING ON THE ENDOCRINE SYSTEM

Steroids Progestogens Oral Contraceptives Thiouracil Sulphonylureas Insulin

SEDATIVES AND ANALGESICS

Barbiturates Dehydrocodeine Pethidine Morphine

TRANQUILLIZERS

Diazepam Chlordiazepoxide Amitryptiline Chlorpromazine Imipramine

MISCELLANEOUS

Chloroquine Indomethazine Metronidazole Paracetamol Salicylates Cytotoxic drugs Prostaglandins

ANAESTHETICS

The effects of anaesthetic agents on the fetus is of itself a large and complicated topic which is properly the province of the anaesthetist. Some cardinal points are set down here. Readers wishing to acquaint themselves with the subject in greater detail are referred to more comprehensive texts.

Volatile anaesthetics. Including ether, chloroform, cyclopropane, halothane, and trilene all cross the placenta, a property no doubt related to their lipoid solubility. Varying times are necessary for equilibration between maternal and fetal circulations, but the interval is quite short. There is thus no reason to expect that, when given for a sufficient time before delivery, they will not produce depression of vital functions in the fetus and provision must be made for adequate resuscitation.

Chloroform is now rarely used in obstetric anaesthesia. Its hepatotoxic action does not seem to be manifest in the fetus.

Cyclopropane has an enhanced depressant effect if acidosis is present as is commonly the case in an infant at delivery.

Local anaesthetics. The ability of local anaesthetics to cross the placenta is poorly documented. It seems that xylocaine may do so.

Basal anaesthetics. Paraldehyde and Chloral both cross the placenta. Bromethol crosses the placenta rapidly and may produce severe respiratory depression in the infant.

Muscle relaxants. Non-depolarizing muscle relaxants such as curare do not cross the placenta although Gallamine may do so in small amounts. Depolarizing muscle relaxants such as succinylcholine cross the placenta poorly.

Atropine. Crosses the placenta and may produce a fetal tachycardia.

ANTIBIOTICS

Penicillins. Penicillins cross the placenta well, as indeed do most antibiotics. Crystalline penicillin will rapidly achieve fetal levels approximating those in the maternal blood. Synthetic penicillins such as Methicillin, Phenethicillin, and Propicillin likewise cross the placenta well.

Ampicillin is perhaps the most useful member of the group as regards pre-natal infection. It crosses the placenta easily and evidence suggests that it is excreted, unchanged and still with anti-bacterial activity, by the fetal kidney into the liquor. This is in turn swallowed by the fetus and thus a reservoir effect is produced. The broad spectrum of activity means that the drug can offer protection against a wide range of organisms, most often unidentified in pre-natal infection at the time of instituting treatment. It attains higher levels in the liquor than in the fetal circulation and is probably the drug of choice in prevention of intrauterine infection. Some workers claim, however, that high dosage to the mother is necessary to maintain a fetal blood level sufficient to give good protection against some strains of E. coli and B. proteus. The low protein-binding activity of ampicillin minimizes the danger of competition for binding sites with bilirubin after delivery. No teratogenicity or other adverse effects on the fetus have been reported with any of these penicillins.

Tetracyclines. Tetracyclines cross the placenta well. They exhibit an affinity for developing bone, in particular the calcifying areas, and the dentine of the developing teeth, where the drug can be demonstrated by fluorescent methods. In animal experiments, interference with bone growth has been shown to occur. In humans, when the milk teeth erupt, these may be discoloured. Although the process is probably reversible and short courses of the drug may not cause much harm, it is best avoided in pregnancy.

Reports about teratogenicity of the tetracyclines are conflicting but in addition to some suspicious case reports in humans, several workers have produced abnormalities, mainly of the limbs, in experimental animals. The incidence of such abnormalities could be reduced by the administration of B vitamins in some series. Such findings would further argue against the use of this group of drugs in potentially or actually pregnant women and if their use is inescapable large doses of B vitamins should be given concomitantly.

Streptomycin. Crosses the placenta well. Large doses in adults are known to produce deafness and in newborns may produce C.N.S. depression also. Although therapeutic amounts given to mothers are unlikely to produce dangerously high levels in the fetus, deafness has occasionally been described in children whose mothers were given the drug during pregnancy. However, the drug is not infrequently given directly to neonates in appropriate dosage, and is a useful therapeutic agent.

Chloramphenicol. In common with other antibiotics this substance crosses the placenta. It is not now commonly used in adults because of the risk of irreversible aplastic anaemia. This complication has not been found in neonates, but in this age group a syndrome of peripheral vascular collapse (the grey syndrome) may occur which can in some cases be fatal. Chloramphenicol acquired across the placenta near term persists longer in the infant's circulation as its breakdown depends on the functioning of liver enzymes, including glucuronyl transferase. For these reasons the drug is obviously to be avoided in pregnancy, but it is a powerful antibiotic and its use may occasionally be mandatory.

CHEMOTHERAPEUTIC AGENTS

Sulphonamides. Animal experiments have suggested that some sulphonamide substances may produce abnormality in the fetus but this has not so far been borne out by clinical experience in the human. These substances may compete with plasma albumin for bilirubin binding sites and thus increase the danger of kernicterus, if given to the newborn and especially the premature baby. As they cross the placenta, sulphonamides should be avoided in women near term for this reason. The long acting sulphonamides are thought to be even more dangerous in this respect owing to their slower rate of excretion.

Trimethoprim. This substance is marketed in combination with a sulphonamide to provide an effective antibacterial drug. Being of low molecular weight it diffuses intra-cellularly with ease and, although there is no experimental work to show that it crosses the placenta, it seems likely that it does so. It has a mild anti-folic acid action which might provide a theoretical reason for caution in its use during pregnancy.

Nalidixic acid. The bulk of evidence derived from animal experiments and studies on pregnant women suggests that this compound is not teratogenic. It is thought to cross the placenta and as it is not metabolized in the fetus (or newborn) in the same way as in older individuals, its use in the last few weeks of pregnancy (and in the newborn baby) is not recommended.

Nitrofurantoin. After a number of years of clinical use, no adverse effects on the human fetus have been reported with this drug. At least one study exists to indicate that it has no such effects. Animal experiments have given similar indications. The drug does not cross the placenta very well and therefore is not suitable for therapy aimed at the liquor amnii or the fetus itself, but, by the same token, is frequently used in treatment of urinary tract infections in pregnancy.

ANTICOAGULANTS

Heparin. Although it is not known for certain whether or not heparin crosses the placenta, the drug appears to have no adverse effect on the fetus if given to the mother.

Coumarol derivatives. Bleeding manifestations in the neonate may occur after therapy to the mother with drugs of this type and these may be fatal. Vitamin K takes some 36 hours to act fully as an antagonist and thus may not be of immediate use. Some cases have indicated that bleeding may also occur in the fetus before delivery.

ANTICONVULSANTS

Barbiturates. See under *Sedatives.*

Phenytoin. Is not under suspicion of being teratogenic having been in widespread use for many years. As with many of the common anticonvulsants, phenytoin is frequently used in combination with other drugs, thus rendering it more difficult to attribute any adverse effects to any one in the regime. Megaloblastic anaemia and thrombocytopenia have been reported occasionally in babies whose mothers have been treated with phenytoin, but this seems to be very rare.

Primidone. This drug crosses the placenta but seems to have no depressant action on the fetus in therapeutic doses. There is little, if anything, to suggest teratogenicity despite its widespread use for many years and animal experiments have yielded no results to contradict this impression.

Ethosuximide. This drug, which is the drug of choice in petit mal epilepsy, is rather poorly documented with regards to its effects on the fetus or placental transmission. The small amount of relevant work does not suggest adverse fetal effects, but is really insufficient to exclude these.

ANTIHISTAMINES

Promethazine. Although marketed originally as an antihistamine, this compound is frequently also used as a sedative. The concensus of opinion indicates that this compound passes rapidly across the placenta. In normal doses for the mother there appears to be no adverse effect on the fetus. Information regarding administration throughout pregnancy is lacking.

Chlorpheniramine maleate. Has been in clinical use for some twenty years without any reports of teratogenic or harmful effects on the fetus, but no definitive experimental work has been carried out.

ANTIHYPERTENSIVES

Guanethidine. This drug does not seem to cross the placenta well. It has been used in pregnant women quite extensively without engendering any suspicion of teratogenicity; nor did experiments with rats indicate any such effect on this species. Evidence does not suggest any other adverse effect on the fetus and the fetal salvage rate is not affected by its use in pre-eclampsia.

Methyldopa. Not much information is available on the use of this drug in pregnancy (although it is quite widely used) or on whether it crosses the placenta, although it probably does. Animal experiments on several species have revealed no teratogenic effect.

Reserpine. Is not as extensively used in hypertension during pregnancy as previously. It does cross the placenta and it is interesting to note that its well known side effect of causing nasal congestion has been observed in neonates following administration to the mother and this may assume clinical importance in terms of airway obstruction.

DIURETICS

Frusemide. This useful diuretic seems to have given rise to no suspicions of teratogenicity in clinical use or in animal experiments. It is playing an increasingly useful role as a diuretic during pregnancy and would be worthy of more intensive study as regards crossing the placenta and the effect on the fetal kidneys.

Chlorthiazide. This and associated thiazide diuretics are presumed to cross the placenta. They are most often used in later pregnancy and in a small number of cases thrombocytopoenia has been observed in the neonate and attributed to these drugs.

HORMONES AND DRUGS ACTING ON THE ENDOCRINE SYSTEM

Steroids. Cortisone and its analogues can certainly induce a high rate of fetal loss and an increased incidence of cleft palate and/or impaired growth in experimental animals. Increased fetal loss and prematurity rates occur in women taking these drugs but there is little real evidence of an increase in the incidence of structural abnormality. It is also difficult to exonerate the disease for which mothers are receiving steroid therapy if the fetus in an individual case is abnormal.

Progestogens. A minority of women who habitually abort appear to suffer from a deficiency of progesterone. It has been suggested that treatment with progestogens may be of value (progesterone itself is ineffective). Although the cases should be selected, e.g. by prior vaginal cytology, and the results are often disappointing, many women have been given such compounds during pregnancy.

1. 19 nor-testosterone, a powerful progestogen, and its close relative norethisterone cause masculinization of the female fetus and for this reason should not be used.
2. 17 α-OH progesterone caproate is less likely to have this effect but it does occasionally occur.
3. Retroprogesterone appears to be the safest of this group from the point of view of masculinizing effects.

Oral contraceptives. The taking of oral contraceptives by a woman who has recently become pregnant has no harmful effect on the fetus as far as can be established.

It has been reported that in pregnancies occurring soon after ceasing oral contraceptives there is a rather higher incidence of abortion and chromosomal abnormalities.

Thiouracil. Thiouracil and its derivatives cross the placenta and frequently produce a goitre in the infant, which in some cases is associated with over- or under-function of the gland.

Sulphonylureas. Tolbutamide and Chlorpropamide both act by stimulating pancreatic secretion of insulin and thus are liable to produce more trouble with hypoglycaemia in the newborn infant. Tolbutamide has been associated with some teratogenic effects in animals and for these reasons, and the fact that insulin can provide much better control and better results in terms of outcome of pregnancy, the sulphonylureas are best not used in pregnant diabetics.

Insulin. Insulin does not cross the placenta. For details of diabetic control and the use of insulin during pregnancy see chapter 8.

SEDATIVES AND ANALGESICS

Barbiturates. This group of drugs in common use have not been reported as likely teratogens. They are known to cross the placenta rapidly but do not seem to have a harmful effect upon the fetus in utero. This is important as it may be necessary to administer these drugs throughout pregnancy, e.g. as anticonvulsants.

There are other important considerations with barbiturates. Firstly, they enjoy widespread use as anaesthetic agents and are known to be respiratory depressants. Owing to their rapid placental transfer, they may produce this effect on the newly delivered fetus. Secondly, it has been found that phenobarbitone has the effect of inducing the enzyme glucuronyl transferase, which is concerned not only with the metabolism of barbiturates but also with the conjugation of bilirubin. Administration of barbiturate to the mother may be of some benefit if severe jaundice is anticipated, although this is not likely to affect the management of hyperbilirubinaemia more than marginally. Thirdly, some recent work suggests that anticonvulsants (and the barbiturates are the most suspect) may interfere with coagulation in the newborn. The defect of coagulation simulates, or may be an exaggeration of, vitamin K deficiency, as prothrombin and factors VII, IX, and X appear to be depressed. Bleeding may occur earlier than the classic haemorrhagic disease of the newborn and is usually, but not always, correctable by vitamin K administration. Barbiturate therapy to mothers may constitute one of the few indications for prophylactic vitamin K given orally to mothers shortly before delivery.

Dihydrocodeine. This drug is useful by virtue of the fact that it has analgesic properties without the severe respiratory depressive actions of the powerful narcotics to which it is related. It has been in widespread clinical use without there being any suspicions of adverse effects on the fetus, either teratogenicity or serious depression of vital functions after delivery. Large doses may produce side effects of a morphine-like nature which can be reversed by the administration of morphine antagonists, e.g. n-allyl normorphine (nalorphine).

Pethidine. This drug is frequently used for sedating parturient women. It crosses the placenta efficiently and may exercise its considerable respiratory depressant effects on the fetus, rendering prompt and expert resuscitation necessary. Its effects may be reversed, like the others in this pharmacological group, by the use of an antagonist. (It is often administered in a combined preparation with an antagonist, e.g. Pethilorfan, in the hope of preferentially suppressing its respiratory depressant effect.) It is a drug of addiction (see also Morphine). Pethidine interferes with heat production from brown adipose tissue, a fact which may sometimes assume clinical importance in the neonate.

Morphine. The use of this drug in labour is best avoided because of its strongly depressant effect on respiration and the ease with which it crosses the placenta to produce this effect in the child. Respiratory depression of the infant is not a problem if the drug is given to the mother within an hour of delivery, but such time is difficult to predict. More appropriate analgesics are usually available. It is a drug of addiction and a fetus chronically exposed to the drug exhibits withdrawal symptoms in the neonatal period.

TRANQUILLIZERS AND MOOD ELEVATORS

Diazepam. This drug is proving very useful in several ways and particularly during childbirth, as it has significant actions as an antidepressive, sedative, and a powerful anticonvulsant. Trials indicate that it may enhance the action of pethidine when the two are used together, but alone does not produce any significant depression of vital activities on the part of the fetus. The drug is known to cross the placenta well, the levels in the fetal circulation being similar, or sometimes higher, than in the maternal circulation; and considerably higher than the levels obtained in the liquor.

Although its deliberate use in pregnant women is mainly during labour and delivery when teratogenicity is not a consideration, its use as an antidepressive may mean that some women will become pregnant while taking the drug. Animal studies have given no hint of a teratogenic effect and in vitro chromosome studies on human embryo cells showed no evidence of its causing chromosomal damage.

Chlordiazepoxide. (See also Diazepam.) In terms of placental passage and teratogenicity studies, this compound behaves much like Diazepam, to which it is closely related chemically.

Amitryptiline. The bulk of information on this compound is derived from animal work which indicates that it crosses the placenta when given in therapeutic doses without adverse effects on the fetuses of the species studied. No case suggesting teratogenicity in the human has been recorded. It should be remembered, if the drug is used at or near delivery, that it potentiates barbiturates.

Chlorpromazine. This and *Promazine* probably do cross the placenta but the amounts appear to be very small.

Imipramine. This compound probably crosses the placenta. On the basis of a fair number of animal experiments, doubts have been expressed about its freedom from teratogenicity although its widespread use in humans has not confirmed this. Like many others, this substance is worthy of further study in this respect.

MISCELLANEOUS

Indomethacin. Teratogenicity studies with animals have shown no such effect of this drug but experience of its use in human pregnancy is lacking.

Chloroquine. Crosses the placenta and achieves high concentrations in fetal tissues. There is no evidence to suggest teratogenicity or other adverse effect on the fetus. Hydroxychloroquine has revealed no teratogenic effect in animal experiments but it is not known for certain how well it crosses the placenta.

However, owing to the chemical similarity of these compounds to quinine, a note of caution might be sounded. The World Health Organisation has suggested a maximum dosage of chloroquine for pregnant women.

Metronidazole. This substance, which is used in the treatment of trichomonas vaginalis infections, crosses the placenta. It has been used during pregnancy without evident damage to the child but more extensive study is required.

Paracetamol. Little definite is known about this drug in relation to whether it crosses the placenta or whether it has any harmful or teratogenic effect. However, the absence of any reports of such effects in a drug which has been so widely used for such a long time might suggest that it is not a teratogen. There is, however, no cause for complacency as drugs of this sort, freely available to the public, ought to be the subject of a thorough investigation and documentation.

Salicylates. Salicylates including acetyl salicylic acid have, in large dosage, produced abnormalities in experimental animals, but there is as yet no convincing evidence that therapeutic doses in man can do so. Although it may not cross the placenta very readily, large doses of salicylate in animals may cause fetal death possibly by poisoning the mother. Congenital intoxication from an intoxicated mother has been described in the human.

Cytotoxic drugs. It might be expected that cytotoxic agents would exert their effects preferentially on the rapidly dividing cells of the developing fetus. This certainly seems true of Aminopterin which has been shown to cause abortion and fetal abnormality when given during the time of organogenesis. The evidence for a similar effect for other cytotoxic drugs is not as convincing. Infants born to women receiving such treatment tend to have low birth weight but the disease process being treated and other therapy probably also play a part in this.

Prostaglandins. Although prostaglandins have not been shown to affect the fetus directly, their influence on uterine activity is of great importance. Prostaglandins $F_{2\alpha}$, and the more potent E_2, when administered intravenously or intravaginally act effectively as abortifacients and will also induce the onset of labour. In the former it is likely they will replace the present techniques, e.g. curettage, vacuum aspiration, hysterotomy etc., with something much safer and in the latter they may well supersede oxytocin. Monthly use of vaginal pessaries might well become a commonly adopted form of contraception. The most troublesome side-effects are vomiting and diarrhoea, which are diminished by using the more powerful fraction and increased if the oral route is used.

Although first discovered in the 1930's, intense interest has only been shown in the past few years. The future involvement of prostaglandins in population control is apparent, but these substances have very many effects throughout the body, and it will be some years before rigorous testing on animals and humans is completed. They are found in many tissues, e.g. lung, spleen, seminal fluid, umbilical cord etc., and have been synthesized chemically. Prostaglandin antagonists have also been produced, e.g. polyphloretin sulphate. As prostaglandin $F_{2\alpha}$ has been found in maternal venous blood during labour, it is tempting to postulate that these antagonists might prevent or inhibit premature labour.

Key references and guides to further reading

BAKER, J. B. E. (1960). 'Effects of drugs on the foetus', *Pharmacol. Rev.*, **12**, 37.

CRAWFORD, S. J. (1965). *Principles and Practice of Obstetric Anaesthesia*, Second edition (Oxford: Blackwell Scientific Publications).

HAGERMAN, D. D., and VILLEE, C. A. (1960). 'Transport functions of the placenta', *Physiol. Rev.*, **40**, 313.

ROBSON, J. M. (1963). 'The action of drugs on the embryo: pharmacological considerations', Section of Experimental Medicine and Therapeutics, *Proc. R. Soc. Med.*, **56**, 600.

SJÖQVIST, F., and UVNÄS, B. (1967). 'Läkemedel och Graviditet', *Nord. Med.*, **78**, 1349.

SMITHELLS, R. W., and MORGAN, D. M. (1970). 'Transmission of drugs by the placenta and breasts', *Practitioner*, **204**, 14.

References

BELMONT, A. P., CHERRY, J. D., and LUCEY, J. F. (1963). 'A lack of relationship between phenothiazine administration to mothers in labor and hyperbilirubinaemia of prematurity', *Am. J. Obstet. Gynec.*, **87**, 538.

BLECHER, T. E., EDGAR, W. M., MELVILLE, H. A. H., and PEEL, K. R. (1966). 'Transplacental passage of ampicillin', *Br. Med. J.*, **1**, 137.

BONGIOVANNI, A. M., and MCPADDEN, A. J. (1960). 'Steroids during pregnancy and possible fetal consequences', *Fertil. and Steril.*, **11**, 181.

BROMAGE, P. R., and ROBSON, J. G. (1961). 'Concentrations of lignocaine in the blood after intravenous, intramuscular, epidural and endotracheal administation', *Anaesthesia*, **16**, 461.

CAVANAGH, D., and CONDO, C. S. (1964). 'Diazepam – A pilot study of drug concentrations in maternal blood, amniotic fluid and cord blood', *Curr. ther. Res.*, **6**, 122.

COHEN, M. M., HIRSCHHORN, K., and FROSCH, W. A. (1967). 'In vivo and in vitro chromosomal damage induced by L.S.D.-25', *New Engl. J. Med.*, **277**, 1043.

EARLE, R. (1961). 'Congenital salicylate intoxication – report of a case', *New Engl. J. Med.*, **265**, 1003.

FLESSA, H. C., KAPSTROM, A. B., and GLUECK, H. I. (1964). 'Placental transport of Heparin', *Clin. Res.*, **12**, 346.

GORDON, R. R., and DEAN, I. (1955). 'Foetal deaths from antenatal anticoagulant therapy', *Br. Med. J.*, **ii**, 719.

Janz, D., and Fuchs, U. (1964). 'Sind antiepileptische Medicamente Während der Swangerschaft Schädlich?' *Dtsch. med. Wschr.*, **89**, 241.

McKay, R. J., and Lucey, J. F. (1964). 'Drugs and the intrauterine and newborn patient', *New Engl. J. Med.*, **270**, 1231.

Monnet, P., Rosenberg, D., and Bovier-Lapierre, M. (1968). 'Thera-peutique anticomitiale administrée pendant la grossesse et maladie hémorrhagique du nouveau-né. Remarques critiques à propos de trois observations personelles', *Rev. franc. Gynec.*, **12**, 695.

Nisbet, R., Boulas, S. H., and Kantor, H. I. (1967). 'Diazepam (Valium) during labour', *Obstet. and Gynec.*, **29**, 726.

Nyhan, W. L. (1961). 'Toxicity of drugs in the neonatal period', *J. Pediat.*, **59**, 1.

Perry, J. E., Toney, J. D., and Leblanc, A. L. (1967). 'Effect of nitro-furantoin on the human foetus', *Tex. Rep. Biol. Med.*, **25**, 270.

Rodriguez, S., Leikin, S., and Hiller, M. (1964). 'Neonatal thrombo-cytopenia associated with antepartum administration of thiazide drugs', *New Engl. J. Med.*, **270**, 881.

Sacks, J. J., and Labate, J. S. (1949). 'Dicoumerol in the treatment of antenatal thrombo-embolic disease', *Am. J. Obstet. Gynec.*, **57**, 965.

Shnider, S. M., and Moya, F. (1964). 'Effects of meperidine on the newborn infant', *Am. J. Obstet. Gynec.*, **89**, 1009.

Staiger, G. R. (1969). 'Chlordiazepoxide and diazepam – absence of effects on the chromosomes of diploid human fibroblast cells', *Mutation Res.*, **7**, 109.

Still, R. M., and Adamson, H. S. (1967). 'Prophylactic ampicillin in the control of intrauterine infection', *J. Obstet. Gynaec. Br. Commonw.*, **74**, 412.

Sutherland, J. M., and Light, I. J. (1965). 'The effect of drugs upon the developing fetus', *Pediat. Clins. N. Am.*, **12**, 781.

Weiss, B. (1959). 'Dihydrocodeine', *Am. J. Pharm.*, 286.

Wilson, M. G. (1962). 'Effect of maternal medications upon the foetus and newborn infant', *Am. J. Obstet. Gynec.*, **83**, 818.

Wren, B. G. (1969). 'Subclinical renal infection in pregnancy', *Med. J. Aust.*, **ii**, 895.

'Symposium on effects of radiation and other deleterious agents on embryonic development' (1954). *J. cell. comp. Physiol.* (Supplement 1), 43.

CHAPTER 8

FETAL INFECTION AND THE EFFECTS OF MATERNAL DISEASE

Maternal infections and the fetus

The newborn infant with an infection may have become infected in utero (prepartum) or during delivery (intrapartum). In utero infection may be acquired by two routes. Firstly, by spread from the maternal blood stream via the placenta, causing widely disseminated, blood borne infection in the fetus, or occasionally via the fetal membranes, when pulmonary infection is common. Secondly, by ascending from the cervix into the amniotic fluid, thence involving the lung, and occasionally infecting the fetus via the placenta. The immunological defence of the fetus before birth depends almost entirely upon maternal IgG antibodies transferred across the placenta, although the fetus produces some IgM antibodies during infection (see chapter 1). Intrapartum infection occurs during passage of the fetus through the birth canal.

INTRAUTERINE INFECTION

Such infections may be viral, bacterial, protozoal or spirochaetal. Any severe maternal infection may cause the fetus to be aborted.

Rubella

Of the viral infections rubella is of the greatest importance because of the teratogenic effects shown in the infected fetus and the possibility of continued virus excretion by the fetus after birth.

Maternal Rubella. The virus is normally spread from the nasopharynx of an infected individual and close contact such as that found in a family is required for passage. It appears probable that an individual can only be infected once since antibodies persist after infection for many years. Infection without a rash does occur in the childbearing years although only in about 10 per cent of cases. Viraemia is present for about seven days before the rash appears and during this time lymphadenopathy is usually present. It has been shown by studies on aborted material that both the fetus and placenta are infected and therefore fetal infection has presumably occurred by the time of the maternal rash. It should be remembered that rubella in-infection may appear very similar to that of measles, scarlet fever or ECHO virus infections.

Pathology. Rubella infection of the fetus causes inhibition of cell growth leading to small overall size and small organs. Destruction of cells also occurs causing loss of parts of formed organs. Different organs seem more affected by infection at different stages of pregnancy and it appears that malformations result from infection during or before the vital time of organogenesis.

Congenital Rubella syndrome. The syndrome has been divided into those cases with congenital defects and an extended or acute disseminated form in which thrombocytopoenia, hepatomegaly, jaundice, bone lesions, etc. may also occur.

The frequency of defects varies in different series, but probably about 20 per cent of neonates show defects when infection occurs in the first four months of pregnancy. The highest defect rate occurs when the mother is infected in the first month, when she may not even be aware that she is pregnant. Maternal infection is also associated with twice the normal abortion and still-birth rate. Multiple defects are found in at least 25 per cent of cases. The incidence of individual abnormalities is given in Fig. 8.1.

The incidence of deafness and visual impairment are in some doubt as these defects are often not immediately evident. Cardiac and eye lesions are associated with first and second

FIG. 8.1. *Clinical manifestations of congenital rubella: percentage incidence of major and minor defects in established cases.* (*Dudgeon, J. A., 1968, Proc. R. Soc. Med.*, 19, *1084*.)

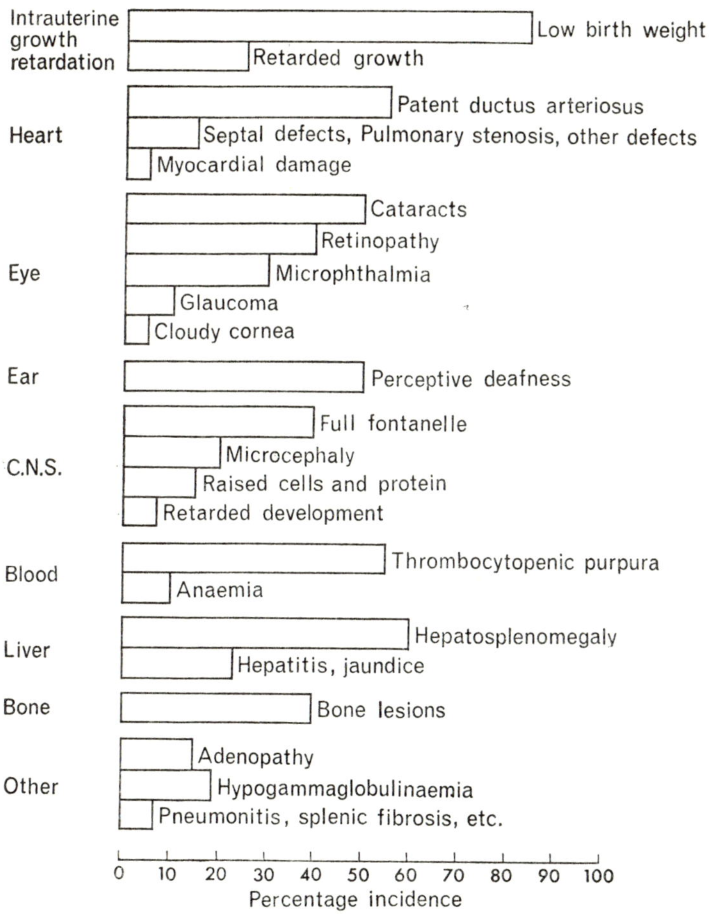

month infection, especially second, and deafness with second, third or subsequent month infection. Deafness from first month infection is usually associated with other defects.

The disseminated type of infection tends to follow infection in the first eight weeks of pregnancy.

Detection of Rubella. Sixty to eighty per cent of infants with congenital rubella have recoverable virus at birth and often excrete virus from the nasopharynx at higher concentrations than infected adults. Ninety per cent at 6 months of age possess neutralizing antibody titres similar or in excess of that of the mother. The presence of antibodies at this time when maternal antibodies have disappeared from the neonatal circulation is good evidence of fetal infection. Abnormally high levels of IgM are present in rubella infants in the first few months of life, presumably produced in response to the intrauterine infection.

In utero rubella infection has been detected by fluorescent antibody studies on amniotic fluid cells.

Maternal rubella infection may be proven by culture of the virus from the nasopharynx and a rising titre of neutralizing, complement fixing and haemogglutination inhibition antibodies.

Prophylaxis by γ-globulin does not seem very effective, presumably because of the low titre of neutralizing antibody to rubella in such preparations.

Cytomegalovirus (C.M.V.)

C.M.V. infection in the adult is usually asymptomatic, so the mother will not know of an infection. Also for this reason it is rarely possible to correlate infection time with the effect on the fetus. The fetus is presumably infected during the time of maternal viraemia, although ascending infection from the cervix is also possible.

Severe congenital C.M.V. infection is characterized by low birth weight, hepatosplenomegaly, microcephaly, mental retardation, motor disability, spastic diplegia, jaundice, choroidoretinitis, and cerebral calcification, but usually only some of the features are present in any one case. Teratogenicity is not shown and the pathological lesions are focal necrosis. As in rubella the virus is excreted in large amounts after birth in the presence of neutralizing antibody. Many affected infants also have IgM levels higher than normal.

Other virus infections

1. Causing fetal death. There is evidence of an increased abortion incidence following maternal infection with measles, mumps, polio, hepatitis, smallpox, vaccinia and influenza.
2. Causing fetal infection. Fetal and placental infection has been shown to occur during maternal infection with measles, varicella, polio, Coxsackie B, smallpox, vaccinia, and possibly herpes simplex. Varicella infection of the mother in the last few days of pregnancy causes a high fetal mortality: necrotic lesions in the skin, intestine and lung of the fetus have been reported. Like the virus of smallpox, the vaccinia virus is very dangerous to the fetus, carrying a high risk of fetal death. During programmes of ring vaccination to contain an outbreak of smallpox, it is probably necessary to vaccinate pregnant women. In all other circumstances, vaccination of pregnant women should be strictly avoided; and it must also be avoided amongst their close family during the pregnancy. Maternal 'hepatitis' has also been associated with neonatal hepatitis, but both C.M.V. and rubella cause neonatal hepatitis.

Tuberculosis

During the immediate post primary tuberculosis or in advanced disease, tubercles may be found in the placenta as a result of haematogenous spread. The fetus becomes infected from these placental tubercles invading the fetal placenta. Haematogenous spread of the disease in the mother does not necessarily mean the fetus will be infected. When the fetus is infected via the placenta tubercle bacilli spread throughout its body, although infection is seen mostly in the liver and lungs. Occasionally infection occurs via the amniotic fluid and membranes, when tubercles are found mostly on the lungs. At birth the infants may appear healthy but rapidly lose weight, develop hepatosplenomegaly and jaundice and die.

Syphilis

Untreated infection of a mother with treponema pallidum may cause transplacental infection of the fetus. If the maternal infection is recent the risk of fetal infection is almost 100 per cent, but the risk decreases to almost nil over the next 10 years in untreated cases. About 25 per cent of infected infants are stillborn and the rest have congenital syphilis. The infants may appear normal at birth but often have fever, restlessness, anaemia and fail to gain weight. The most common findings are a maculopapular rash (like that of adult secondary syphilis), mucocutaneous lesions, condylomata lata, severe rhinitis ('snuffles') due to nasal ulceration; and hepatosplenomegaly, sometimes with ascites and oedema. Bone lesions are common and low grade meningitis may be present. Later manifestations include gummata, periostitis, keratitis, deafness, rhagades, abnormal teeth and neurosyphilis. Diagnosis may be made by finding the spirochaetes on dark ground illumination of scrapings from moist cutaneous lesions. Tests based on antibodies are of no use in the first six months of life, if the mother is seropositive, as such antibodies in the infant will be of maternal origin.

Toxoplasmosis

Toxoplasmosis when acquired by the mother is usually subclinical except for perhaps a few enlarged lymph nodes. Serological testing shows that the disease is common. The fetus may be infected from the mother via the placenta during maternal infection and the toxoplasmas distributed throughout the fetal body. Toxoplasmosis shows a predilection for nervous tissue producing disseminated meningoencephalitis and choroidoretinitis. Hepatosplenomegaly with jaundice and lymphadenopathy are common. Many affected infants are stillborn and most live born fetuses have low birth weights. Subsequent pregnancies are not affected. The disease may be detected by patchy calcification in the brain on a skull X-ray but such findings are not always present in the neonatal period.

Listeria

Listeria monocytogenes infection in the adult may be mild and asymptomatic. The fetus is often stillborn with hepatitis, purpura, and multiple granulomata in many organs, or liveborn with meningoencephalitis. Intrapartum infection also occurs causing meningoencephalitis. The organisms may be isolated from the maternal vagina and sometimes from the urine and blood.

Malaria

Pregnancy, especially in the latter months, may cause severe exacerbation of malaria even when the condition is latent. With high fever and rigors the incidence of abortion and premature labour is greatly increased. Even when treatment is instituted the fetal loss is still high. It is said that malaria cannot pass through a normal placenta but merozoites may enter the fetal circulation during delivery.

URINARY TRACT INFECTION

Asymptomatic bacteriuria

The presence in two successive fresh clean midstream urine samples of more than 100,000 bacteria per ml is termed asymptomatic bacteriuria and is an indication that organisms are multiplying in the urinary tract. The level of bacteriuria is assessed by colony counts and for this dip inoculum tests are now widely used. Such bacteriuria is present in 3–7 per cent of pregnancies and is commoner in lower social class groups. Up to 40 per cent of affected women develop urinary tract infection in later pregnancy. Reports that bacteriuria is associated with prematurity, hypertension, pre-eclampsia, and high perinatal mortality have not been confirmed. (The incidence of bacteriuria in non-pregnant women of childbearing age is also about 5 per cent.)

Pyelonephritis

This condition is associated with an increased fetal loss by abortion, premature labour, and intrauterine death due to hyperpyrexia.

INTRAPARTUM INFECTIONS

Infections associated with birth affect mostly the skin and eyes, by direct contact of these with infected areas in the birth canal, and the lungs, by inhalation of infected amniotic fluid or of material in the vagina, during delivery.

Pneumonia

In most cases infection is associated with ascent of vaginal organisms into the uterine cavity after rupture of the membranes. Such infection is commonly associated with histological evidence of placentitis and the presence in the fetal lung of neutrophil polymorphs showing multilobed nuclei, presumably of maternal origin. (Fetal polymorphs usually show only one or two lobes.) Factors predisposing to such infections are:

1. Premature rupture of membranes.
2. Prolonged labour from any cause, with or without early rupture.
3. Obstetric manipulation.

The rate of infection is considered high 24 hours after rupture of membranes. The organisms involved are most often coliforms and Staph. aureus but Klebsiella, Pseudomonas, and Proteus are relatively common. Because of the risk of infection 24 hours after rupture of the membranes, prophylactic antibiotic therapy is required. The drug must have a wide spectrum of activity and be concentrated in the amniotic fluid, hence ampicillin is mostly commonly used. If ampicillin is given after 24 hours and delivery takes place within three days ampicillin should be administered to the infant. If the rupture to delivery interval is longer than three days, a different antibiotic should be given to the infant.

The lungs may also become infected by inhalation of organisms in vaginal mucus and debris during delivery.

Skin. Neonatal skin sepsis caused by staphylococci and candida albicans may be contracted during delivery or soon after delivery.

Eye. Infection of the eye from contact with gonocci during delivery, although once a common cause of blindness, is now rare. Many 'sticky' eyes in neonates have no obvious infective cause although staphylococci and viruses, e.g. T.R.I.C. and C.M.V. virus, have been implicated. Such infections may well be acquired after birth.

Maternal disease

Many severe diseases are associated with a low incidence of pregnancy and a high abortion and still-birth rate.

Any muscular or skeletal disease or anomaly may affect the fetus by causing prolonged and difficult labour. Often the fetus is delivered by elective caesarean section for this reason.

DISEASES ASSOCIATED WITH AUTOANTIBODIES

Idiopathic Thrombocytopoenia Purpura (I.T.P.)

The role of IgG anti-platelet antibodies as an aetiological factor in I.T.P. is now widely accepted. The perinatal mortality rate amongst infants born to mothers with I.T.P. is about 16 per cent and thrombocytopoenia is a large factor in this mortality. About half of liveborn infants have clinical and haematological features of I.T.P. which resolve over the first 12–16 weeks of life (the time course of IgG denaturation). Maternal treatment for I.T.P. has no effect on the fetal condition at birth.

Thyrotoxicosis

L.A.T.S. (Long acting thyroid stimulus) has been demonstrated in the case of thyrotoxic patients and has been considered to be IgG antibody. It has also been found in the serum of infants with neonatal thyrotoxicosis and their thyrotoxic mothers. This suggests placental transfer of L.A.T.S. causing the neonatal disorder.

Myasthenia Gravis

The possibility that myasthenia gravis is an autoimmune disease is based largely on the presence in the serum of some cases of antibodies to striated muscle. About 20 per cent of infants born to mothers with this disease show some features of neonatal myasthenia gravis. These are hypotonicity, respiratory and feeding difficulty, and a feeble cry. Antibodies to muscle striations have been demonstrated in some of these infants.

Anticholinesterase therapy during pregnancy may also be a cause of neonatal myasthenia. Drugs such as pyridostigmine may be slowly eliminated from the body and cross the placenta. In the fetus high doses of the drug may cause neuromuscular blocking leading to fetal weakness and necessitating anti-cholinesterase therapy.

HEART DISEASE IN PREGNANCY

Congenital heart disease

Maternal congenital lesions usually have little effect on the well-being of the fetus. Rarely, in cases of severe pulmonary hypertension or large right-to-left shunts, perinatal mortality is increased due to fetal hypoxia causing intrauterine death or premature labour. Normal spontaneous vaginal delivery is allowed and induction of labour or caesarean section are employed for purely obstetric reasons. However, in cases of aortic coarctation caesarean section may be advised because of the small risk of rupture of the aorta or an associated berry aneurysm.

Rheumatic heart disease

The incidence of this disease is diminishing, and in general, with good management, pregnancy in such cases is uneventful. Careful assessment of cardiac status must be made early in the pregnancy. Because of effective treatment of cardiac failure and the minimization of the risk of bacterial endocarditis by antibiotic cover for instrumental delivery or intrauterine manoeuvres, the risk to the mother of therapeutic abortion is the same as that of delivery. If indicated valvotomy may be performed during pregnancy with little effect on the fetus. Pregnancy has also been successful in patients with prosthetic heart valves.

There is evidence of salt and water loss in infants born to women having intensive diuretic therapy, but this is not clinically detectable.

HORMONAL AND METABOLIC DISORDERS

Diabetes

The management of pregnancy in a diabetic woman poses three main problems:

1. Pregnancy causes difficulty in control of maternal diabetes.
2. Diabetes increases the incidence of many complications of pregnancy.
3. The unusual environment for the fetus results in a high rate of stillbirth and of death and morbidity in the neonatal period.

Although the untreated diabetic is subfertile, with adequate treatment fertility is normal. When pregnant the outcome of her pregnancy is independent of the duration of diabetes or the mode of treatment used before pregnancy. However, the control of diabetes during pregnancy and the vascular and hypertensive sequaelae of the disease have a profound effect on the well-being of the fetus.

The fetus of a diabetic mother is exposed to higher sugar, fatty acid and ketoacid levels than normal. As ketoacids cross the placenta and high levels have a very detrimental effect on the fetus, maternal ketoacidosis must be avoided.

The weights of infants of diabetic mothers are commonly high. However, when maternal blood sugar levels are well controlled infants of normal weight may be born. Another reason why an infant may have normal weight is the antagonistic effect of maternal hypertension and pre-eclampsia upon the tendency to high birth weight. High birth weights are considered due to the high glucose load to which the fetus is subjected, hyperglycaemia causing pancreatic β-cell hypertrophy, high fetal blood insulin levels and consequent high fat deposition. At birth the baby often has a moonface, coarse bloated features, and hirsuties giving the appearance of Cushing's syndrome.

The fetus of a diabetic woman is usually delivered prematurely and commonly suffers from respiratory distress syndrome. A high incidence of congenital abnormalities is reported in diabetic pregnancies. Neonatal hypoglycaemia is common and is believed to be associated with hyperinsulinism. It certainly seems that such infants have high insulin levels at birth and that they reduce the blood sugar level after an oral glucose load more rapidly than normal infants. Both hypoglycaemia and high birth weight may be associated with the high adrenal cortical activity and low adrenaline secretion which have been found in these infants.

The need to control blood sugar levels during pregnancy when calorie intake must be maintained and the renal threshold is low means that very little reliance should be placed on urinary sugar levels. A good calorie intake is required to prevent carbohydrate starvation and its consequent ketoacidosis. Oral hypoglycaemic agents are best avoided and are associated with neonatal hypoglycaemia (see chapter 7). Some substances, e.g. placental lactogen found in the serum in pregnancy, exert an anti-insulin effect and may be partly responsible for changes in diabetic control.

For all these reasons the diabetic mother should have an ample diet and frequently requires to be treated with insulin, controlled by frequent blood sugar estimations, although some diabetics may still be managed by diet alone.

Diabetic pregnancy may be complicated by pre-existing hypertension and by a high incidence of pre-eclampsia. Other problems are a large infant, the need for induction of labour and the increased incidence of polyhydramnios and uterine inertia.

Management of diabetic pregnancy

A glucose tolerance test (G.T.T.) should be performed for any of the following indications:

1. A family history of diabetes.
2. Previous delivery of a large baby.

3. Previous unexplained stillbirth or neonatal death.
4. Glycosuria on more than two occasions.

Glycosuria of diabetes must be distinguished from renal glycosuria of pregnancy, which has not been convincingly shown to be a danger to the fetus. Renal glycosuria occurs because the renal threshold for glucose is reduced from 180 to 120 mg/100 ml or less. This is probably related to the increased glomerular filtration rate which occurs in pregnancy, together with unchanged tubular reabsorption of glucose.

In the normal G.T.T. the fasting blood sugar (venous blood) should not exceed 110 mg/100 ml, and no value should be more than 160 mg/100 ml. After two hours from the start of the test the blood sugar level should be back to normal. Corresponding capillary blood values are 120 mg/100 ml and 180 mg/100 ml.

Because of the lowered renal threshold for glucose, large quantities of carbohydrate are lost into the urine, predisposing to ketosis. Also as a result of the altered threshold, routine urine-testing for sugar becomes unhelpful as a method for diabetic control. The clinician must rely on blood sugar estimations despite inconvenience to patient and laboratory.

The maternal demand for insulin increases in pregnancy, and the extra amounts required may be considerable. It is often possible to maintain good control with a once-daily injection of insulin using a mixture of quick- and slow-acting insulins, altered according to the blood sugar values. In order to obtain better stabilization it is often necessary to administer the insulin twice daily. It is common practice, near term, to convert entirely to soluble insulin therapy giving three or four injections daily. This is not always necessary if the blood sugar levels are monitored frequently from early pregnancy, with adjustments of the insulin dosage as needed. Serial blood sugar levels are estimated three- or four-hourly starting early in the morning, with the patient having her normal diet, and performing usual activities as far as possible. The blood samples are taken during the waking hours only, and a profile of blood sugar levels is obtained. From this the clinician can easily see in which part of day adjustment of insulin dosage is required. The usual diet should contain 150–180 g of carbohydrate, and should also be altered, as necessary, to produce steady control of blood sugar levels. These should be kept between 100 and 150 mg/100 ml.

Traditionally diabetic patients have been admitted to hospital from the 30th or 32nd week (until delivery) for stabilization of the diabetes. Using the methods described above it should be possible to reduce the amount of in-patient treatment, restricting admission to those women in whom stabilization is difficult to achieve, or who develop pre-eclampsia.

Where control has been good, delivery can be delayed until the thirty-eighth week. In adequately controlled diabetes, there should be a reduced incidence of hydramnios, of pre-eclampsia, and the babies should not be abnormally large. Delivery should be by the vaginal route if possible. Surgical induction by amniotomy is performed and an oxytoxic intravenous infusion is set up at the same time. Caesarean section, once the favoured method of delivery, can be reserved for cases where labour is not quickly established, where progress is slow, and where there are obstetric indications for it.

During labour, sufficient glucose must be given by the intravenous route to cover the insulin and prevent ketosis. After delivery the requirements for insulin decrease immediately and the patient can be given two-thirds of the pregnancy dosage. Further blood sugar estimations may be necessary to re-stabilize the diabetes in the puerperium.

When elective caesarean section is planned, this should be a joint procedure involving obstetrician, anaesthetist, and paediatrician. Depending on the time of day chosen, the pre-operative insulin dosage is usually reduced, and glucose given by intravenous drip.

Myxoedema

Although uncommon in childbearing years this condition is associated with subfertility, loss of libido, and frequently abortion. With treatment pregnancy is normal.

Disorders of the adrenal cortex

Fertility is decreased in Cushing's syndrome as amenorrhoea is a common feature of this disease. Patients taking steroid treatment for Addison's disease, late onset adrenogenital syndrome or after adrenalectomy for Cushing's disease, if the dosage is large at term, may cause suppression of the neonatal adrenal, although this is rare.

Phenylketonuria

Adequate treatment of phenylketonuria means that such individuals are now reaching childbearing years. The fetuses of such women are at risk from maternal high phenylalanine levels even though the fetus itself may be free of the disease. Therefore low phenylalanine diets have been recommended for these women during pregnancy. The fetus is possibly also at risk during pregnancy of women with 'atypical' phenylketonuria or heterzygous for the condition.

HAEMATOLOGICAL DISORDERS

Iron deficiency

The mother transfers 250–400 mg of iron to a single fetus. If maternal iron stores are depleted, even if there is no anaemia, the fetal stores are lower and the fetus may develop anaemia in the first year of life.

Folate deficiency

Maternal anaemia due to folate deficiency becomes manifest in later pregnancy. Severe anaemia is associated with a high perinatal mortality rate. It is reported that a high percentage of patients with abruptio placentae have signs of folate deficiency but there are also contrary reports. Epileptic mothers treated with phenytoin, phenobarbitone, or primidone run a greater risk of folate deficiency.

Haemoglobinopathies

Sickle cell anaemia and sickle cell-haemoglobin C disease are both associated with pre-eclampsia and high fetal loss although less so in the latter disorder. The low birth weight found in infants of women with sickle cell disease is thought possibly due to blood stasis in the placenta secondary to sickling. Sickle cell trait has no ill effect on the fetus or the pregnancy.

β-thalassaemia causes a blood film appearance similar to iron deficiency even though iron stores in this condition are often very high and iron therapy contra-indicated. Patients with this condition run a higher risk of folate deficiency during pregnancy.

Leukaemia and Hodgkin's disease

X-ray therapy may be carried out during pregnancy except in the first trimester. Adequate shielding of the fetus is essential. The use of cytotoxic drugs is probably best avoided and is contra-indicated in the first trimester as they have been shown to cause congenital malformations when given during the time of organogenesis. Forty per cent of infants born to mothers having such treatment have low birth weights.

SURGERY DURING PREGNANCY

Surgical procedures should not be performed during pregnancy unless there is no alternative treatment, or where other measures have failed.

There is an increased chance of abortion, premature labour, deep vein thrombosis, and pulmonary embolism, and intra-uterine death associated with surgery and the pyrexia of post-operative infection. The risk appears less between the third and eighth months. Adequate pre-oxygenation should be given, and where the operation is abdominal, minimal handling of the uterus is essential. Intramuscular injections of progesterone derivatives have been administered in an attempt to suppress uterine contractions, but are probably of little effect. The use of beta-adrenergic inhibitors, e.g. isoxsuprine hydrochloride, may be more effective.

Operations may have to be performed for the following reasons during pregnancy:

Ovarian cystectomy   Appendicectomy   Cholecystectomy Strangulated hernia Ruptured spleen (traumatic or spontaneous) Intestinal obstruction Thyroidectomy Orthopaedic and general trauma.

Mitral valvotomy Closure of patent ductus Resection of coarctation of aorta.

Craniotomy for intra-cranial tumours.

Biopsy of cervix.

This list is by no means comprehensive.

Clearly the operations for thyrotoxicosis, gall bladder disease, and rheumatic heart disease, are only carried out where medical treatment has failed, and the mother's life is in danger. Thanks to the efficacy of modern drug therapy these operations are rarely necessary. In the literature, descriptions of almost every cardiac operation can be found, including the use of the cardio-pulmonary bypass with extra-corporeal circulation.

Ovarian cysts are usually detected at the first ante-natal clinic visit. They should be removed because of the dangers of torsion, obstructed labour, and for histological examination because of the high risk of malignancy. It is usual to wait until after the 16th week by which time the placenta is functioning and there is less chance of abortion. If found in the last trimester it is wiser to wait until term. If, after labour starts, the cyst impacts in the Pouch of Douglas, then caesarean section and ovarian cystectomy should be performed. On the other hand, if labour is not obstructed, then laparotomy should be undertaken early in the puerperium and the cyst removed. Torsion is common in the puerperium.

The maternal mortality from acute appendicitis increases toward term, and the abortion and prematurity rates increase with the presence of complications, e.g. pelvic abscess and peritonitis. Diagnosis is often difficult due to the displacement of the appendix upwards and outwards, and surgery may be delayed. There appears to be a reduced ability in pregnancy to wall-off infection. This is probably due to poor access to the omentum due to the enlarged uterus, Braxton-Hicks contractions preventing adhesions, increased vascularity and lymphatic drainage, and increased corticosteroid production. Fetal loss is overall about 12 per cent, but may be over 50 per cent where peritonitis has developed.

Cone biopsy of cervix should be carried out in pregnancy, where a positive cervical smear has been obtained, despite the dangers of haemorrhage and premature labour. It is clearly important to distinguish between dysplasia, carcinoma-in-situ, and invasive carcinoma. Definitive treatment of invasive carcinoma is carried out immediately in early pregnancy, but if detected later, treatment can be delayed until after delivery. Wedge and punch biopsies of visible lesions can also be performed during pregnancy.

PRE-ECLAMPSIA

Although an enormous amount of research has been carried out into the hormone, enzyme, electrolyte, and immunological changes, in this condition, the exact aetiology is still far from clear. The disease is characterized by hypertension, oedema, and albuminuria; the first of this triad forming the basis of the diagnosis. Many clinicians diagnose pre-eclampsia on the presence of hypertension and one of the other two signs, after the 20th week. In attempting to define the disease, one finds there is no general agreement about what the normal and abnormal blood pressure in pregnancy should be. Most obstetricians take 140/90 as hypertensive, but many are now accepting the lower level of 130/80 as the upper limit of normal. The presence of oedema alone cannot indicate pre-eclampsia as over 60 per cent of all pregnant women develop the sign, which seems to be of no pathological significance. Albuminuria is also unhelpful as it only appears where the pre-eclampsia is severe.

Whilst pre-eclampsia occurs in 25 per cent of primigravida, it also occurs in association with other abnormal situations of pregnancy, e.g. diabetes mellitus, multiple pregnancy, hydramnios, rhesus iso-immunization, and hydatidiform mole. A few cases turn out to be cases of essential hypertension making its first clinical appearance during pregnancy, although this is usually decided in retrospect. Pre-eclampsia may well be a group of disorders.

The reader is referred to more comprehensive sources of information dealing with the aetiology and bodily changes that have been observed. He will note the conflicting opinions, and differing laboratory results.

As far as the fetus is concerned there is an increased perinatal mortality. Small-for-dates babies occur, and there are increased still-birth and first-week death rates. The effects on the fetus appear to be due to reduced placental blood flow with subsequent impairment of nutrition. The lesion causing this is an acute fibrinoid necrosis of the maternal arteries in the placental bed. This is later followed by a lipophage infiltration. It is extremely interesting to note that similar pathological changes have been observed in the renal arteries of rejected kidney transplants. It has therefore been suggested that the fetus is rejecting the mother, and not vice-versa as has also been proposed. Such ingratitude has yet to be immunologically verified.

Treatment of the condition is empirical. It consists of improving the placental blood flow, and delivery of the fetus when it is mature, if possible. A careful balance must be made between the detrimental effects of the pre-eclampsia and the equally lethal disadvantages of prematurity. The majority of cases occur during the last six weeks of pregnancy, and admission to hospital is usual. Bed rest is the only known way of improving placental blood flow. Mild sedatives are also usually given, but it is only in the severer grades of pre-eclampsia that the anticonvulsive properties of the barbiturates and other drugs are required. The use of hypotensive drugs has not been shown to improve fetal survival, and even in severe cases, are ineffective in preventing or controlling eclamptic fits, when used alone.

Excessive weight gain has been considered to be an early sign of pre-eclampsia, and for many years low-salt and low carbohydrate diets have been inflicted on unwilling patients in an attempt to make them lose weight. The apparently beneficial effects of such management, obtained over thirty years ago, was undoubtedly due to attention to detail. The patients were examined frequently in ante-natal clinics, pre-eclampsia was diagnosed early, and admission to hospital arranged if necessary. In other words, they had proper ante-natal care. It now seems that such dieting may not only be valueless but actually dangerous, and obstetricians are now far more concerned about weight *loss*, particularly when there is hypertension. (See 'Increase in weight and girth,' chapter 3.)

Similarly the weight loss produced by diuretics may be confusing. Although these drugs will reduce oedema, there is no evidence that they improve fetal survival.

The well-being of the fetus can be monitored by serial total oestrogens or oestriol estimations, though this is probably unnecessary in cases of mild pre-eclampsia of short duration. All cases should have frequent blood-pressure recordings, examinations of the urine for albumin, and weighings. Induction of labour by amniotomy is performed as near to term as possible depending on the response to bed rest and sedation. Where the condition is not controlled despite treatment, and where there is persistent albuminuria, delivery should be effected regardless of the maturity of the fetus. In pre-eclampsia, persistent albuminuria, and prolongation of the pregnancy beyond term are both lethal factors affecting fetal survival.

Separation of the placenta (accidental haemorrhage, abruptio placentae) which is one of the maternal complications of pre-eclampsia, has an extremely high stillbirth rate – over 50 per cent. Immediate caesarean section may improve the chances of survival but this is not usually feasible as the fetus is often already dead, or the mother severely shocked.

The reader is again referred elsewhere to standard textbooks, for details of the complications of pre-eclampsia, separation of the placenta, and renal failure.

ESSENTIAL HYPERTENSION

This is diagnosed if the pregnant woman is found to have a raised blood pressure before the twentieth week, and where no underlying cause for it has been found.

Mild uncomplicated cases of essential hypertension have similar perinatal mortality rates to those of uncomplicated pre-eclampsia. Unfortunately where pre-eclampsia is added to an existing essential hypertension, the mortality rates are very much higher.

Where the hypertension is moderate to severe (diastolic >100 mmHg), it is usual to exclude other causes of hypertension, e.g. coarctation of the aorta, phaeochromocytoma, chronic glomerulonephritis, or chronic pyelonephritis etc. The patient is admitted to hospital, and a full general examination is carried out, if not already done. A mid-stream urine is sent for bacteriological examination and tested for albumin, a 24-hour collection of urine is examined for excess of catecholamines, and renal function tests are performed. These include blood urea and creatinine clearance estimations. Where chronic renal disease exists with severe impairment of renal function, termination of pregnancy may be indicated. In less severe cases, the renal function tests can be repeated at intervals, and if these show a deterioration later in the pregnancy, premature delivery of the baby may be indicated. This is because of the high stillbirth rate, and also because of the deleterious effect on the maternal renal function. Phaeochromocytoma cases are in such jeopardy from left ventricular failure, hypertensive crises, and placental separation, that surgical removal should be undertaken regardless of the length of gestation.

The management of essential hypertension is much the same as for pre-eclampsia. Hypotensive therapy generally has been disappointing in terms of fetal survival, and is usually reserved for the more severe grades. In women in the later years of reproductive life, with a long history of hypertension and a blood pressure of 180/110 mmHg, the prognosis for the fetus is poor, and these patients will require long periods of hospitalization for rest. Hypotensive drugs may be indicated, and monitoring of the fetus as for pre-eclampsia is essential to guide the obstetrician as to the optimum time for delivery.

A pregnancy complicated by pre-eclampsia may hasten the onset of permanent essential hypertension in a woman destined to develop it later in life. However, it is not thought that pre-eclampsia actually causes it. Moreover, pre-eclampsia does not appear to cause any chronic renal disease. There seems to be a familial tendency to pre-eclampsia, which is unrelated to a hypertensive diathesis.

References and guides to further reading

BARNES, C. G. (1970). *Medical Disorders in Obstetric Practice*, Third edition (Oxford: Blackwell Scientific Publications).

BLACKHALL, M. I., BUCKLEY, G. A., ROBERTS, D. U., ROBERTS, J. B., THOMAS, B. H., and WILSON, A. (1969). 'Drug-induced neonatal myasthenia', *J. Obstet. Gynaec. Br. Commonw.*, **76**, 157.

BLAIR, R. G. (1963). 'Phaeochromocytoma in pregnancy', *J. Obstet. Gynaec. Br. Commonw.*, **70**, 110.

CORNBLATH, M., PILDES, R. S., and WARRNER, R. A. (1970). 'Infants of diabetic mothers', *Early Diabetes*, eds. Camerini-Davalos, R., and Cole, M. S. (New York: Academic Press).

DIXON, H. G., and BRANT, H. A. (1967). 'The significance of bacteriuria in pregnancy', *Lancet*, **1**, 19.

DUDGEON, J. A. (1967). 'Maternal rubella and its effect on the fetus', *Archs. Dis. Childh.*, **42**, 110.

—— (1968). 'Virus infections of the human fetus', *Proc. R. Soc. Med.*, **19**, 1084.

JONES, W. R. (1967). 'Immunological diseases and pregnancy', *Br. J. Hosp. Med.*, **1**, 718.

MACGILLIVRAY, I. (1969). 'Hypertension in pregnancy', *Modern Trends in Obstetrics*, 4, ed. Kellar, R. J. (London: Butterworths).

NICHOLSON, H. OLIPHANT (1968). 'Leukaemia in pregnancy', *J. Obstet. Gynaec. Br. Commonw.*, **75**, 517.

PEDERSEN, J. (1967). *The Pregnant Diabetic and her Newborn* (Copenhagen: Munksgaard).

ROBERTSON, W. B., BROSENS, I., and DIXON, H. G. (1967). 'The pathological response of the vessels of the placental bed to hypertensive pregnancy', *J. Path. Bact.*, **93**, 581.

WADE, G., NICHOLSON, W. F., and MORGAN JONES, A. (1958). 'Mitral valvotomy and pregnancy', *Lancet*, **1**, 559.

YU, J. S., and O'HALLORAN, M. T. (1970). 'Children of mothers with phenylketonuria', *Lancet*, **1**, 210.

CHAPTER 9

GENETICS AND GENETIC COUNSELLING

Introduction

In man the genetic code is carried in the nuclear deoxyribonucleic acid (D.N.A.). This D.N.A. is present as long helical double filaments in the chromosomes. The sequence of nucleic acids in these D.N.A. strands determines the nature of the cell proteins and hence the structure and function of the cell.

Normal cells contain 23 chromosome pairs comprising 44 somatic and 2 sex chromosomes; this is termed the diploid number of chromosomes. The gametes contain half this number of chromosomes (22 somatic and 1 sex chromosome) and are termed haploid.

The genes of the genetic code are paired because the chromosomes are paired and thus there are two sets of information for any given trait, such as, the presence or absence of a red cell antigen or an enzyme in a metabolic pathway, or the number of fingers. If each of the genes in a pair hold the same information for a certain trait, the individual is termed homozygous for this trait, and if the genes of the pair hold different information then heterozygous for the trait. When a heterozygous individual exhibits a trait for which the information is carried in only one of the gene pair, then that gene trait is dominant and the genetic information not expressed is recessive. For the information of a recessive gene to be expressed the individual must be homozygous for that gene.

The outward expression of genetic information is called the phenotype and the underlying genetic constitution the genotype. In a heterozygous individual a dominant gene causes the phenotype to express a given trait although the genotype possesses both dominant and recessive gene information. Thus in the heterozygous state the phenotype and genotype are different.

DOMINANT PATHOLOGICAL TRAITS

Dominant pathological traits tend to be less severe than recessive conditions. If a dominant trait causes such a severe disorder that reproduction is impossible, it will disappear, whereas a recessive condition, although often lethal when homozygous, may not be so in the heterozygous state and may even confer an advantage thus becoming more widely disseminated. A person showing a dominant trait is therefore usually heterozygous and will normally mate a homozygous individual free of the pathological gene.

Unless the abnormal dominant gene appears by a new mutation, it will usually be seen in each previous generation. Although the chance of each child of an affected parent inheriting the disease is 50 per cent, the percentage of affected offspring in any family differs from this because of random variation.

DOMINANT PATHOLOGICAL CONDITIONS

Skeletal: Achondroplasia (most cases), multiple exostoses, osteo-genesis imperfecta.

Muscular: Muscular dystrophy (facioscapulohumeral), myotonia congenita, myotonia dystrophica, peroneal muscular atrophy.

Nervous: Huntingdon's chorea, neurofibromatosis.

Haematological: Elliptocytosis, spherocytosis.

Other: Diabetes insipidus (vide infra), epidermolysis bullosa

FIG. 9.1. *Inheritance of a dominant pathological trait.*

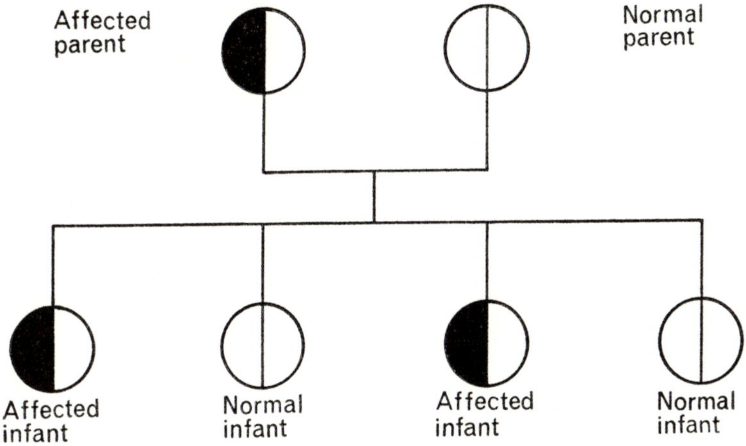

simplex, hyperelastosis cutis, multiple polyposis of the intestine, polycystic kidneys, acute intermittent porphyria, variegate porphyria.

RECESSIVE PATHOLOGICAL TRAITS

The abnormal trait due to a recessive gene is only expressed when the individual has both genes of the gene pair as the recessive abnormal type. The normal gene is dominant over the abnormal gene and thus the heterozygote has a normal phenotype. In the mating of two heterozygous individuals the chance of any infant being affected is 25 per cent.

Two phenotypically normal people may therefore produce an affected infant, and in addition there may be little or no family history of the condition. It should be noted that the absence of a family history does not necessarily exclude a genetic cause for an abnormal trait. The chances of mating two heterozygous individuals is statistically very low.

FIG. 9.2. *Inheritance from parents heterozygous for an abnormal trait.*

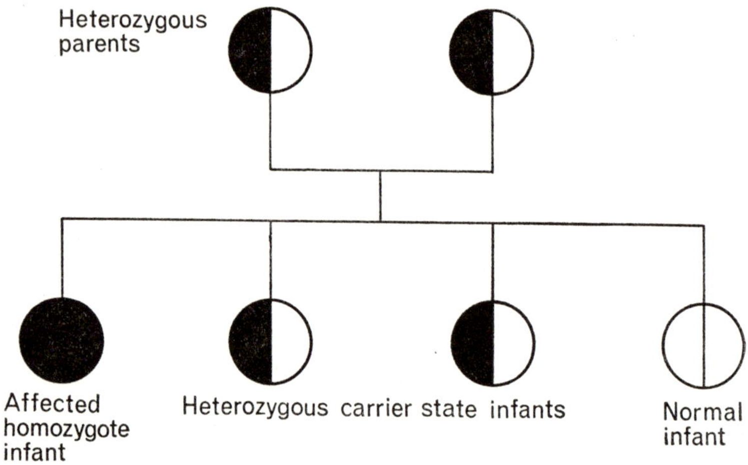

For example, the frequency of the abnormal gene for galactosaemia is about 1 : 200 and the overall incidence 1 : 40,000, but as the abnormal gene is present in only a few families, mating within these families gives a very much higher incidence of the disease.

The mating of a homozygous person demonstrating an abnormal recessive trait with a heterozygous normal individual gives a risk for any infant being affected of 50 per cent and the same risk for the carrier state.

An individual homozygous for an abnormal trait mating a homozygous normal individual will have no affected infants but all of them will be carriers.

The mating of two individuals homozygous for an abnormal trait results in all infants being affected.

RECESSIVE PATHOLOGICAL CONDITIONS

Muscular: Muscular dystrophy (limb girdle type), pro-

FIG. 9.3. *Inheritance from one parent homozygous (affected) and the other heterozygous for the same condition.*

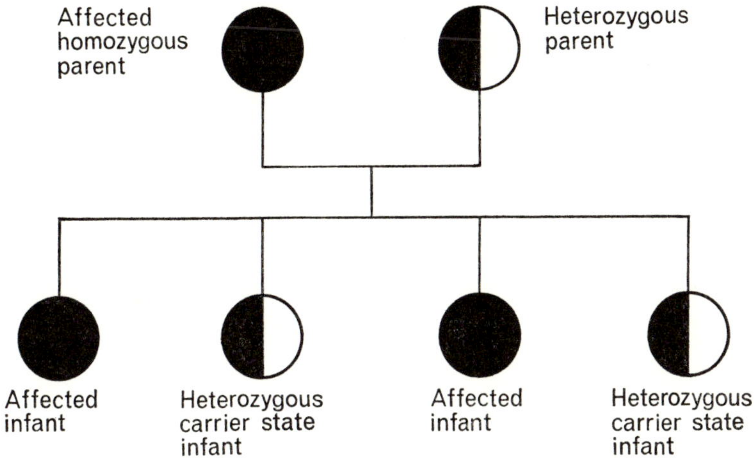

gressive spinal muscular atrophy (Werdnig-Hoffman), peroneal muscular atrophy.

Nervous: Friedrich's ataxia, Tay Sach's disease.

Hormonal: Adrenogenital syndrome, familial goitrous cretinism.

Metabolic: Albinism, alcaptonuria, cystinuria, hereditary fructose intolerance, galactosaemia, most mucopolysaccharidoses, several glycogen storage diseases, Hartnup disease, Wilson's disease, hypophosphatasia, phenylketonuria.

Other: Cystic fibrosis, microcephaly, Niemann-Pick's disease, sickle cell anaemia, thalassaemia major.

SEX LINKED RECESSIVE PATHOLOGICAL TRAITS

The female possesses two X chromosomes and the male one X and Y chromosome. The X chromosome carries many genes for normal body function, such as colour vision, whereas the Y

FIG. 9.4. *Inheritance from homozygous normal and homozygous affected parents.*

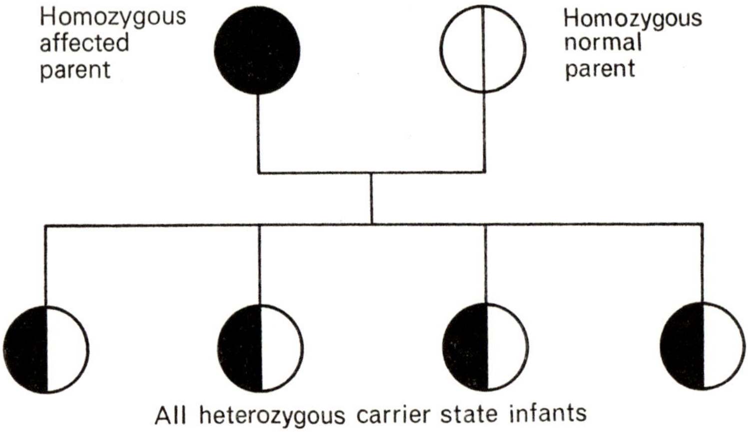

chromosome is concerned mostly with maleness. Thus the X genes in the male are largely unpaired and an abnormal gene on the X chromosome will be expressed even if recessive.

In the mating of a female carrier of a recessive abnormal trait on the X chromosome to a normal male the risk of an affected male child is 50 per cent and similarly the risk of a female carrier-state child.

The mating of an affected male with a homozygous normal female results in normal male offspring and carrier state female offspring. Half of the male children of this female offspring will exhibit the abnormal trait. In this fashion recessive sex linked disorders often appear to miss generations and are seen in propositus and grandfather.

A female carrier mating an affected male results in half the male infants being affected and half normal, and half the female infants being affected and half carrier-state. Thus a female may exhibit a sex-linked recessive disorder if the condition is common

FIG. 9.5. *Inheritance from normal male and carrier state heterozygous female parents.*

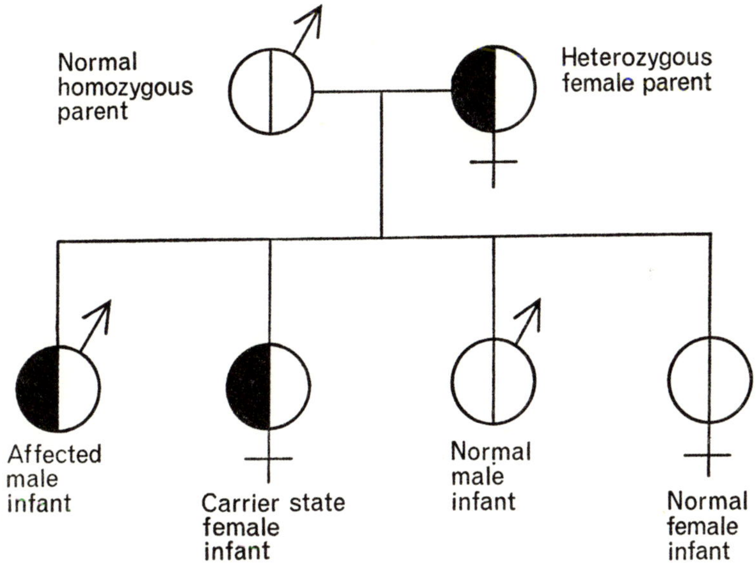

or in consanguineous marriages. For instance, the mating of a haemophiliac male with a carrier-state female may result in a haemophiliac female child.

SEX LINKED RECESSIVE PATHOLOGICAL CONDITIONS

Haemophilia, Christmas disease, colour blindness, Hunter's syndrome (mucopolysaccharidosis II), muscular dystrophy (Duchenne type), peroneal atrophy, glucose-6-phosphate dehydrogenase deficiency.

Further comments

In the lists of genetic disorders it will have been noted that some diseases appear in more than one group. Because these diseases have more than one mode of inheritance it is very important to obtain a full family history so that the mode of inheritance in any particular case may be judged with a view to adequate genetic counselling. Some examples of variation of inheritance of related diseases are given below. Although 7 out of 8 cases of achondroplasia are transmitted in an autosomal dominant fashion, 1 in 8 is sporadic and there is no family history of the disorder. Of the mucopolysaccharidoses, types I, III, IV, V, VI (McKusick) are transmitted by autosomal recessive genes and type II (Hurler's) is a sex-linked recessive disorder. The muscular dystrophies show all three main modes of inheritance: the facioscapulohumeral type and dystrophica myotonica are autosomal dominants, the limb girdle type is an autosomal recessive and the Duchenne type is sex-linked recessive. The inheritance of nephrogenic diabetes insipidus is almost certainly autosomal dominant, but although most of the inherited pituitary diabetes insipidus are also autosomal dominant, some are sex-linked recessive. Similarly Swiss type thymic alymphoplasia is inherited as an autosomal recessive but there is a sex-linked variant.

MODIFICATIONS OF THESE MECHANISMS

The standard models of genetic inheritance of simple gene pair abnormal traits are in reality often greatly modified in their expression by genetic and environmental factors.

Genetic. Some pathological traits depend on more than one pair of genes so that a genetic disposition may only be expressed in the presence of other genetic abnormalities. The association of hare lip and cleft palate is of this type. Occasionally dominant traits appear to skip generations. In this way an apparently normal individual may transmit an abnormal trait to his offspring. Careful examination of this individual may reveal a slight abnormality and the gene is then deemed to have reduced expressivity. In some cases the reduced defect may be tested for, e.g. red cell fragility in hereditary spherocytosis or skeletal X-ray examination for multiple exostoses.

When no expression of the gene is found, the skipping of a generation is termed reduced penetrance in that generation.

Incompatibility of genetic factors may cause reduced gene expression. This is commonly seen in Rhesus iso-immunization when cells from a Rhesus positive fetus do not cause antibody formation in the Rhesus negative mother because of ABO blood group incompatibility (see chapter 6).

Another modification of the normal mechanisms is shown in thalassaemia. In this condition the homozygous state known as thalassaemia major is a lethal disorder with a large percentage of the circulating haemoglobin as HbF. The heterozygous state has a slight increase in HbF levels, runs a variable, usually benign, course and is known as thalassaemia minor. In many other recessive conditions, the heterozygous state shows a mild abnormality normally only detectable by biochemical means (vide infra).

Environmental. Certain hereditary diseases only become manifest under unusual environmental conditions. For instance, glucose 6 phosphatase dehydrogenase deficiency only becomes apparent when the individual is exposed to fava beans, primaquine, sulphonamides etc. Similarly acute intermittent porphyria is often made apparent by the administration of barbiturates; and pseudocholinesterase deficiency when suxamethonium is used as a muscle relaxant during general anesthesia.

ABNORMAL CHROMOSOMES

About 1 per cent of infants at birth have a chromosomal anomaly. Of these less than a quarter reach maturity. Identification of an abnormal chromosome pattern is important as regards the prognosis of the affected infant and genetic counselling of the parents.

Peripheral blood cells or cells from tissue biopsy may be cultured in nutrient media. After 72–96 hours of culture, colchicine is added to stop cell division in metaphase, when the nuclear membrane has dissolved. The cells are osmotically ruptured and the chromosomes fixed, stained, and photographed. Alternatively they may be identified by autoradiographic labelling of replication. From the photograph the chromosomes can be paired and the pairs placed in their groups according to size and shape. (Note: The chromosomes appear as two chromatids joined by a centromere which, had cell division continued, would become two separate chromosomes.) Abnormal numbers of chromosomes and chromosomes with absent or extra parts may then be noted.

TABLE 9·1 *Some common chromosome abnormalities*

Condition	*Chromosome number*	*Sex chromosomes*	*Abnormal chromosomes*
Normal male	46	XY	
Normal female	46	XX	
Kleinfelter's syndrome	47	XXY	Extra X
Turner's syndrome	45	X	Absent X or Y
Trisomy 18 (male)	47	XY	Extra 18
Trisomy 13 (male)	47	XY	Extra 13
Down's syndrome			
Trisomy 21	47	XY	Extra 21
Translocation	46	XY	18/21 translocation

Another anomaly detectable by chromosome studies is that of mosaicism. A mosaic is an individual with cell lines, or tissues, of different chromosome numbers. Obviously many cells or tissues must be studied before mosaicism can be diagnosed with certainty.

GENETIC COUNSELLING, INTRODUCTION

Genetic advice is sought from two sources. Firstly, the parents of an abnormal child wishing to know whether they should have further children and, secondly, a person having a close relative with a genetic defect wishing to know the risk of any of their children having this defect. The advising physician should inform the parents of the consequences of a genetic abnormality, whether it is treatable, and the risk of offspring having the abnormality. The decisions of the parents will be based not only on the physician's advice but also on religious, social and emotional factors.

EXCLUSION OF NON-GENETIC CAUSES

Many congenital defects do not have an inherited genetic cause. For instance, fetal defects caused by rubella or toxoplasmosis may mimic genetic disorders. A careful history of the relevant pregnancy and consequent studies on the infant must be taken with special reference to the general state of health, medication, and irradiation of the mother during the time of fetal organogenesis. It must be remembered that not all genetic conditions show themselves at birth. Conditions such as Huntingdon's chorea or Friedrich's ataxia are not manifest till some years after birth and thus the birth of apparently normal infants does not exclude these disorders.

FAMILY PEDIGREE

This is a time-consuming process but of great importance in assessing the mode of inheritance of any defect. The information obtained is best plotted on a pedigree chart. Questions should be asked to obtain information regarding numbers of individuals in previous generations, those individuals with the defect or anything resembling the defect, miscarriages, and stillbirths, causes of death, consanguineous marriages, illegitimacy, and adoption. From this information it is usually possible to judge the mode of inheritance of any defect, allowing for the modifications mentioned previously. Great care must be taken with those diseases having multiple forms of inheritance.

DETECTION OF THE HETEROZYGOUS STATE

Just as incomplete expression of a dominant gene causes minor genetic abnormalities so may heterozygotes for some recessive pathological conditions express minor defects. Most frequently these abnormalities are regarded from an academic viewpoint after the birth of an affected infant. However, if there is a family history suggesting a possible carrier state an individual may seek advice and suitable tests may be undertaken. For instance the female carrier state for haemophilia tends to have a lower factor VIII level than normal. The heterozygous state of phenylketonuria shows abnormal phenylalanine tolerance. An individual carrying the gene for some of the mucopolysaccharidoses often shows abnormal incorportion of radioactive sulphur into the mucopolysaccharides of fibroblast cultures.

SOME DISEASES IN WHICH THE HETEROZYGOTE MAY BE DETECTED

Autosomal condition	*Abnormal finding in heterozygote*
a β-lipoproteinaemia	Abnormal lipoprotein electrophoresis
Anophthalmia	Small eyeballs
Congenital afibrinogenaemia	Low plasma fibrinogen
Cystic fibrosis	Abnormal sweat test and metachromasia in fibroblast cultures
Galactosaemia	Decreased red cell levels of galactose-1-phosphate uridyl transferase
Glycogen storage disease (type III)	Decreased leucocyte amylo-1,6-glucosidase
Haemoglobinopathies	Abnormal haemoglobin electrophoresis
Mucopolysaccharidoses (some forms)	Abnormal sulphur incorporation into fibroblast cultures
Histidinaemia	Decreased skin histidase
Phenylketonuria	Abnormal phenylalanine load test
Pseudoxanthoma elasticum	Angioid retinal streaks
Xeroderma pigmentosa	Excess freckling

SEX-LINKED

Condition	*Findings in carrier-state female*
Glucose-6-phosphate dehydrogenase deficiency	Decreased red cell glucose-6-phosphate dehydrogenase levels
Haemophilia	Decreased levels of antihaemophilic globulin (A.H.G.)
Muscular dystrophy (Duchenne type)	Increased serum creatinine phosphokinase (C.P.K.).

DETECTION OF MODIFIED GENETIC DEFECTS

As has been mentioned above some dominant pathological traits may not be apparent because of reduced expressivity and may be detected by biochemical or radiological means.

PARENTAL GENOTYPE

This is of particular use in assessment of the risk of Rhesus incompatibility. Because of the easy access to the red cell antigen and the availability of specific antisera, the parental genotypes for the Rhesus antigens may be assessed with some certainty and therefore the risks of a further affected fetus more accurately decided.

RISK OF AFFECTED OFFSPRING

This is most easy to assess when the disease is known to be controlled by a single gene.

1. Autosomal dominant (e.g. Huntingdon's chorea). The chance of any given infant having the disease if one parent is affected is 50 per cent.
2. If a child is born showing a recessive trait (e.g. phenylketonuria) the risk of another infant being affected is 25 per cent.
3. If an affected male for a sex-linked recessive abnormality (e.g. haemophilia) mates with a normal female the male offspring will be normal and the females will be carriers.
4. If a carrier-state female for a sex-linked recessive condition marries a normal male, 50 per cent of the males will be affected and 50 per cent will be normal, and of the females 50 per cent will be carriers and 50 per cent normal.

Very many conditions have less certain modes of inheritance; for instance, mental deficiency, epilepsy, spina bifida, and hydrocephalus.

RISK OF AFFECTED INFANTS IN SOME OTHER CONDITIONS

Mental deficiency of unknown origin. The risk of an affected sibling to a mentally retarded propositus depends on whether the parents are affected.

Statistical data indicates the following:

Both parents normal	15 per cent chance of further affected infant
One parent defective	35 per cent chance of further affected infant
Both parents defective	90 per cent chance of further affected infant

Mongolism (21 trisomy). The overall frequency is about 1 in 700 births. In women under 30 years of age the incidence is 1 in 2,000 and in those over 45 years 1 in 54.

Anencephaly. Where one infant shows this abnormality the risk to the subsequent child is 1 in 30, and the risk of spina bifida is the same. If two infants are anencephalic the risk is greatly increased.

Spina bifida alone. The risk to further siblings, if there is one affected child, is 1 in 25 for spina bifida and for anencephaly, but 1 in 9 if there are two affected children.

Hare lip. The chances of subsequent children showing this abnormality appears independent of whether cleft palate is also present. There is a 1 in 20 risk to siblings of an affected child born of normal parents. The risk to any infant born of a parent having hare lip is 1 in 50, but if the abnormality is also present in a sibling then 1 in 10.

Cleft palate alone. The risk to a sibling of an affected propositus born of normal parents with no affected close relatives is 1 in 80, but if a first degree relative shows the abnormality the risk is 1 in 10.

Mosaicism. Where it has been established that a parent is a mosaic, the risk of an infant inheriting an abnormality depends solely on genetic constitution of that parent's gonads.

CONTRACEPTIVE ADVICE

Where appropriate, opportunity to discuss contraception often occurs in connection with genetic advice. Parents of children with hereditary disorders, who feel the risk of further affected children is unacceptable, are not always willing to ask advice concerning contraception. The discerning physician, being aware of this, will inform the parents where such advice may be obtained.

References and guides to further reading

BARTALOS, M. (1968). *Genetics in Medical Practice* (London and Lippincott: Pitman).

CLARKE, C. A. (1964). *Genetics for the Clinician* (Oxford: Blackwell).

EVANS, D. A. PRICE (1965). 'The detection and significance of heterozygotes in neurometabolic disorders', *Biochemical Approaches to Mental Handicap in Childhood* (Edinburgh and London: E. and S. Livingstone).

HSIA, D. Y. (1966). *Inborn Errors of Metabolism*, Part I, Second edition (Chicago: Year Book Medical Publishers).

ROBERTS, J. A. FRASER (1963). *An Introduction to Medical Genetics*, Third edition (London: Oxford University Press).

CHAPTER 10

MANAGEMENT OF FETAL ABNORMALITIES

Obstetric management

In the not-too-distant future it is very likely that the in utero detection of fetal abnormalities will be reliable and comprehensive. Biochemical and cytogenetic techniques used early in pregnancy may allow the clinician and his patient sufficient time to consider therapeutic abortion as a solution to the problem of an abnormal fetus. It is also possible that some metabolic disorders may be 'treated' in utero. However, as most of these studies have been carried out on amniotic fluid, it is highly unlikely, in the light of present knowledge and experience, that all pregnancies will be tested.

Procedures to detect fetal abnormalities would be used in various 'at risk' conditions, e.g.:

1. Pregnancy with polyhydramnios, oligohydramnios or failure to increase uterine size.
2. Women with an obstetric history of certain types of abnormality, e.g. spina bifida.
3. Women with a family history of certain types of abnormality, e.g. a mucopolysaccharidosis.
4. Perhaps in elderly women because of high incidence of mongolism.

In traditional obstetric practice it is probably true to say that very few fetal abnormalities are detected before delivery, and, excepting those which may cause mechanical obstruction during labour, they are of little importance as far as labour-ward management is concerned.

Hydrocephaly when present may be severe enough to prevent engagement of the fetal head in the maternal pelvis. It may be detected by abdominal palpation in the last trimester, and confirmed by X-ray examination. Minor degrees are not incompatible with vaginal delivery, but where cephalo-pelvic disproportion exists, perforation of the distended fetal head by means of a spinal or similar needle, may be necessary. Cerebrospinal fluid is released and the head collapses. This is usually performed during labour through the dilating cervical canal. When the breech is presenting in such an infant, the after-coming head can be tapped. If there is an associated spina bifida, the head can be collapsed by passing a catheter into its opening and up into the cranium.

Occasionally the condition is not diagnosed until labour has started. On vaginal examination, the cranial sutures and fontanelles are felt to be wide. Radiological examination during labour, viz. abdominal and erect lateral pelvic views, may be indicated, if there is any difficulty in deciding whether cephalo-pelvic disproportion is present.

Anencephaly rarely causes any problem in labour, but occasionally there is difficulty in the delivery of the shoulders. The classical physical sign is hydramnios which is present in over 50 per cent of cases. Hydramnios can also be associated with other congenital abnormalities, e.g. oesophageal atresia, spina bifida, hydrocephalus, cleft palate, congenital heart disease etc. Occasionally, especially where anencephaly is present, hydramnios may cause such discomfort to the patient, e.g. pain, dyspnoea, oedema of the legs and feet, that amniocentesis is necessary. A suitable cannula is used, and the amniotic fluid is released slowly to lessen the likelihood of placental separation. Enough fluid is removed to make the patient comfortable. If a standard 'drip set' is used, controlled release can be effected. It cannot be over-emphasized that an X-ray of the maternal abdomen must be requested in every case of hydramnios. Major skeletal abnormalities can be detected and multiple pregnancy excluded. After delivery, in cases of hydramnios of unknown aetiology and where the baby appears externally normal, a tube should be passed into the stomach to exclude oesophageal atresia, which is surgically correctible.

Where twin pregnancy has been diagnosed careful attention should be paid to the attitude of the two fetuses. Although unusual, where the fetal heads lie exactly alongside each other conjoined twinning should be suspected. Delivery by caesarean section may be preferred.

Radiological examination may also show microcephaly or limb deformities such as those seen in achondroplasia or phocomelia, but these do not cause difficulties in delivery.

X-ray or ultra-sonic cephalometry may be of additional assistance in the diagnosis of minor degrees of hydrocephalus. Intra-amniotic injection of Myodil, which outlines the fetal trunk, may demonstrate the presence of a meningomyelocele as a break in the continuity of the dye along the fetal back.

Where a fetal abnormality has been detected, the clinician must decide whether to inform the patient herself, or the husband only. This decision must take into account the emotional state, the intelligence, and suspicions, of the patient. Many obstetricians induce labour when the diagnosis has been made. Others allow labour to start spontaneously wishing to avoid the risk of a caesarean section for failed induction where there is a grossly abnormal baby. Happily induction of labour, employing amniotomy, and oxytocin drip is largely successful. Except in cases of disproportion, every effort should be made to obtain a vaginal delivery in such cases.

In utero detection of metabolic and chromosome disorders

The prenatal detection of genetic disorders, both biochemical and chromosomal, increases the precision of genetic counselling since one has evidence of the abnormality in the fetus itself. The growth of such studies has expanded largely due to the increased use of amniocentesis and the ability to culture amniotic fluid cells of fetal origin.

The timing of amniocentesis is important. This procedure is difficult before twelve weeks of gestation and of increasing ease after this time. Methods requiring culture of amniotic fluid cells are subject to a delay due to the time taken to grow the cells (about 20–30 days until the second subculture). This may mean that if amniocentesis is not undertaken early the fetus is about twenty weeks when abortion is considered, with the ensuing unpleasantness.

SEX DETERMINATION

This is of immense value where there is evidence of an X-linked disease, e.g. haemophilia or Duchenne muscular dystrophy. Both nuclear sexing and chromosome karyotyping have been used to determine this. The absence of Barr-bodies in amniotic cells obtained by abdominal puncture may be shown in frozen sections prepared from the cells. Such a technique is sufficiently rapid that the cells may be examined in an anteroom and the clinician may then, on the result, proceed to hysterotomy if required.

DETERMINATION OF CHROMOSOMAL ABNORMALITIES

Chromosome analysis of cultivated amniotic fluid cells has been used to show Down's syndrome in the fetuses of women known to be carriers of D/G translocation. Such methods may be employed in any case where the woman or her husband have been shown to have an inheritable chromosome abnormality. Some workers use chromosome analysis for sex determination.

DETECTION OF RED CELL ANTIGENS

The ABO blood group of the fetus may be determined by testing fetal amniotic fluid cells. Reports of Rhesus grouping by these techniques have not been confirmed.

BIOCHEMICAL STUDIES IN CULTURED AMNIOTIC FLUID CELLS

Enzyme assay. The list of enzymes which have been demonstrated in amniotic fluid cells increases rapidly. The absence of enzymes has allowed pre-natal detection of many diseases including galactosaemia, Hunter's syndrome, and Tay-Sach's disease. Information obtained from studies of this nature, besides allowing opportunity for abortion of affected fetuses, enable the clinician to commence treatment of diseases such as galactosaemia at birth.

Metachromasia. Amniotic cell cultures from fetuses having Hurler's or Hunter's syndrome have shown metachromatic staining with toluidene blue and an increased rate of radio sulphur incorporation.

BIOCHEMICAL STUDIES DIRECTLY ON AMNIOTIC FLUID

Enzyme activity. Enzyme activities have been measured on direct assay of amniotic fluid cells, thus dispensing with the time delay of cell culture. Cells must be obtained before twenty weeks as cells taken after this time have a low activity.

Steroid estimations. Increased 17-oxogenic steroids and pregnanetriol levels in amniotic fluid near term have been shown to be helpful in diagnosing congenital adrenal hyperplasia at about 39–40 weeks. This allows treatment of the condition to be commenced at birth.

Bilirubin. Measurement of amniotic fluid pigment in blood group iso-immunization is discussed in chapter 6.

BIOCHEMICAL STUDIES ON MATERNAL URINE

Consistently low oestriol levels in maternal urine in the third trimester in the absence of anencephaly have been of value in allowing the diagnosis of adrenal cortical hypoplasia to be made before birth.

Low urinary oestriol levels in association with normal pregnanediol excretion is highly suggestive of anencephaly.

A NOTE OF CAUTION

It should be remembered that amniocentesis is not without risk and that the rate of successful culture of amniotic fluid cells is not 100 per cent even in the most skilled hands (some workers now report about 90 per cent success).

Many of the methods mentioned above are not widely used and require great skill on the part of laboratory workers. The clinician should therefore be sure that the results obtained from the laboratory are accurate and reproducible and that adequate positive and negative controls are used in biochemical and histochemical studies. In general these more difficult methods should be considered as still in the stage of development.

References and guides to further reading

ABBO, G., and ZELLWEGER, H. (1970). 'Pre-natal determination of fetal sex and chromosomal complement', *Lancet*, **1**, 216.

CATHRO, D. (1969). 'The adrenal cortex and medulla', *Paediatric Endocrinology*, ed. Hubble, D. (Oxford: Blackwell Scientific Publications).

EDWARDS, J. H. (1970). 'Uses of amniocentesis', *Lancet*, **1**, 608.

FRATANTONI, J. C., NEUFELD, E. F., UHLENDORF, W., and JACOBSON, C. B. (1969). 'Intrauterine diagnosis of the Hunter and Hurler syndromes', *New Engl. J. Med.*, **280**, 686.

LENNON, G. G. (1967). 'Intra-uterine foetal visualization', *J. Obstet. Gynaec. Br. Commonw.*, **74**, 227.

NADLER, H. L. (1968). 'Antenatal detection of hereditary disorders', *Pediatrics*, **42**, 912.

——, and GERBIE, A. B. (1969). 'Enzymes in non-cultured amniotic fluid cells', *Am. J. Obstet. Gynec.*, **103**, 710.

Report of Scientific Meeting at the Royal College of Obstetricians and Gynaecologists (1966). 'Foetal malformation', *J. Obstet. Gynaec. Br. Commonw.*, **74**, 455.

CHAPTER 11

PRE-NATAL ENVIRONMENTAL INFLUENCES ON BEHAVIOUR

JOHN H. W. BARRETT
B.A., B.Sc.
Department of Psychology
University of Bristol

Introduction

At birth, Chinese children are a year older than their European peers. The European convention for assigning age implicitly ignores the pre-natal period, and may well have encouraged the fashion for assuming that between conception and birth there can occur little or nothing of psychological importance. However, there are more compelling reasons for the neglect within science, though not within folklore, of intrauterine behavioural influences.

A number of commonly held assumptions have tended to inhibit research. For example, it has often been assumed that individual differences in behaviour apparent at birth are mainly genetically determined, that the fetus is largely protected from environmental influences, and that, in any case, the fetal nervous system is insufficiently developed to register experience. Such assumptions have remained tenable until recently as a result of a number of empirical factors, which have themselves tended to discourage research. First, pre-natal influences on behaviour are often swamped by pre-natal influences on morphology, and by post-natal child-rearing and social-class variables. Second, techniques for *in utero* monitoring of fetal responses have been primitive, unreliable and difficult to use. Third, there has been a healthy reluctance to disturb mother or fetus for purposes of research. And fourth, there has been a scarcity of information on the neurophysiological and endocrinological mechanisms which might mediate influences on behaviour.

Current research findings, however, strongly question these assumptions. Highly controlled work on animals, which will be discussed more fully in the next section, has shown clear evidence of pre-natal non-genetic transmission of information (Denenberg, 1969). Further, it has shown that almost any treatment applied to a pregnant animal results in differences of some kind between her offspring and those of untreated controls, and has led to the suggestion that the protection from external stimuli which the fetus is accorded by the womb is largely offset by its extreme sensitivity (Joffe, 1969).

The assumption that the fetal nervous system is unlikely to register experience requires slightly more detailed discussion, as it depends in part on a series of assumptions, most of which have been challenged by recent neurophysiological findings. It has often been assumed, for example, that the cerebral cortex does not begin to function until some months after birth. It has long been known that the cortex is largely unmyelinated at birth, and often assumed that unmyelinated tracts are non-functional. Superficial comparisons of the responses of the human neonate and the anencephalic infant served to reinforce the conclusion that the neonate, and therefore the fetus, was indeed non-functional at a cortical level. However, myelination is not necessary for conduction. Even 'myelinated' fibres can conduct long before the morphological appearance of myelin, and although myelination is accompanied by lower thresholds, shorter latencies, higher amplitudes, and increased conduction velocities, conduction times in the fetus can be faster than in the adult owing to the shorter paths involved (Timiras et al, 1968).

Corroboration comes from recent E.E.G. studies. E.E.G. activity has been recorded from the human fetus from an

Estimated Conceptual Age (E.C.A.) of seven weeks onward, which is before the development of the primitive grey matter, and this reinforced the assumption that the fetal E.E.G. is of sub-cortical origin. However, Weitzman et al (1968) recorded intrinsic E.E.G's and auditory evoked responses in all the premature infants they studied, including some of E.C.A. 23 weeks, and considered that some components were of cortical origin. Further, even in their most premature subjects, E.C.A. 24 weeks, Hrbek et al (1970) found visual and somato-sensory evoked responses which were most prominent over the corresponding projection area, and concluded that they reflected actual cortical events. Whether these findings apply in utero remains to be elucidated; other studies, however, indicate that the E.E.G. activity of prems and of fetuses of the same E.C.A. is very similar. The characteristics of these early E.E.G's differ in many ways from those of more mature subjects, and amongst other things reflect the differing degree of myelination, but it seems clear that there can be considerable real cortical activity by about the beginning of the second half of fetal life, if not earlier.

However, in addition to these demonstrations of the possible functional relevance of the cortex, earlier developing sub-cortical mechanisms probably play a more significant role, particularly at earlier fetal ages (Bergström, 1969). Further, neuronal activity as such is unlikely to be as significant in the mediation of early influences on the development of behaviour as the chemical processes it reflects. Environmental influences operate profoundly through such chemical variables as nutrition, oxygen supply, and hormones, and in this connection it is likely that the mechanisms of metabolic adaptation (McIlwain, 1970) will prove to be of particular importance. (The implications of metabolic adaptation will be discussed further in section 4.)

Both as a tissue and as an organ, the brain is characterized by the plasticity of its reponses to change in the internal and external environment, and the especial vulnerability of the developing brain has frequently been emphasized (Timiras et al, 1968). The behavioural syndromes which accompany easily detectable morphological anomalies brought about by environmental influences have been discussed frequently and comprehensively elsewhere. Although the distinction is necessarily arbitrary, this chapter will concentrate on pre-natal variables which influence post-natal behaviour without obvious morphological effects. It will be seen that there is now a substantial body of data on the effects of various pre-natal influences on such aspects of behaviour as activity level, emotional responsivity, personality type, attention, intelligence and ability, and on such disorders of behaviour as the 'colicky child syndrome'. As a leader in the British Medical Journal put it in 1964, the uterine environment may give rise to subtle changes which, 'though causing no macroscopic abnormality, may somehow affect those developing neural tissues of the fetus which govern behaviour in later life'.

1. Some implications of the animal studies

Before discussing in more detail the influences on the human fetus, it will be valuable to take a brief and cautious look at the implications of some of the animal studies. Caution is necessary because, as Fraser (1964) pointed out in relation to teratogenesis, extrapolation from animals to man 'is unwarranted unless supported by evidence in man'. The need for caution has been explicitly underlined by many of the animal studies themselves: it is a frequent finding that influences and effects are not only species-specific but also strain-specific. The many animal studies have recently been comprehensively reviewed by Joffe (1969). Here, attention will be confined to a few of the more general implications of the animal work, and to a few examples of important recent findings.

In many ways the findings have themselves vindicated the value for human studies of experiments on pre-natal influences in animals. Rigorous controls and experimental manipulations have begun to unravel the complex interactions of large numbers of pre-pregnancy, pre-natal and post-natal variables, whose significance must usually remain masked or unreplicated in the inevitably more or less uncontrolled human studies. Further, use of the rat and other animals with relatively large litters and short inter-generation times, has made it possible to control, manipulate, and trace influences across several successive generations, and thus uncover mechanisms which, even were rigorous control possible, would probably take centuries to demonstrate in man.

The pre-natal variables which have been shown in rat studies to have significant post-natal effects include nutrition, oxygen, radiation, drugs, herbicides and pesticides, hormones, population stress and overcrowding, sound, handling, and psychological stresses such as fear or anxiety. The range of offspring behaviours affected is also wide, and includes motor performance, activity level, exploration, emotionality as measured in the open-field test, mating behaviour, and various forms of learning, including olfactory discrimination and maze and avoidance learning.

It is of particular importance when implications for man are being considered that large and significant post-natal effects are frequently produced by manipulations which, superficially at least, would appear to be of a minor if not subtle nature. The manipulation known as 'handling' is an example. The standard form of this treatment merely involves the animal being taken from its home cage, held in the experimenter's hand for three minutes, and then replaced in the cage. The treatment is typically carried out once daily over a period, for example throughout pregnancy, or from birth to weaning. Many studies have shown handling once daily through pregnancy to have significant effects on offspring behaviour, even when the offspring have been fostered by non-handled mothers. Other studies have shown significant effects of pre-natal maternal handling on offspring physiological and biochemical variables. Ader and Deitchman (1970), for example, have demonstrated it can significantly accelerate the maturation of the offspring's diurnal adrenocortical rhythms.

Handling need not be merely pre-natal to have significant

effects, it can be pre-mating. In elaborate and well-controlled studies, it has been found (Denenberg et al, 1963, 1968) that mothers who were handled for three minutes daily for the first 20 days of life produced offspring which at weaning at 21 days were significantly more emotional and less active in the open-field test than the offspring of non-handled controls. Parallel physiological studies (Levine, 1967) found significantly lower plasma corticosterone levels at weaning in the offspring of mothers handled during their own infancy, together with a significantly reduced response to novel stimulation. Thus, infantile handling influences the as yet unconceived generation. Other studies have shown that effects on offspring behaviour can result from experiences such as anxiety undergone by the mother in adulthood but before mating. And Joffe's (1969) demonstration that maternal experience in maturity, as well as in infancy, can influence offspring behaviour both pre-natally via the uterine environment and post-natally, via rearing behaviour, is of great methodological importance.

The influence of environmental variables such as handling is persistent. Using appropriate controls, Denenberg and Rosenberg (1967) found that infantile handling significantly influenced the emotionality and open-field behaviour of grand-pups, and thus demonstrated what they described as the 'non-genetic transmission of information' across three generations. It appears (Denenberg, 1969) that such 'granny effects' may operate either through the uterine environment or through maternal behaviour or through both. (In man such long-term 'granny effects' are frequently confounded by much more direct 'mother-in-law effects'!) Other non-genetic 'granny effects' have been shown by Ressler (1966) who produced significant differences in the visual exploration behaviour of mice reared by their own parents simply by manipulating the strain of their foster-grandparents. Likewise, Wehmer et al (1970) found that conditioned anxiety during pregnancy increased the activity and reduced the emotionality (open-field test) of the grandpups. They concluded that infantile handling, anxiety before pregnancy and anxiety during pregnancy can each influence the behaviour of future generations beyond the immediate offspring.

Perhaps enough has been said to indicate that the recent animal studies have already demonstrated much that in the not so distant scientific past might well have been dismissed as superstition. The methodological implications of the animal work will be further discussed in the next section.

The main substantive findings can be summarized thus:

1. In some mammals environmental events during pregnancy can alter the intrauterine environment and, without obvious morphological effects, influence offspring behaviour.
2. The range of maternal experiences and treatments during pregnancy which can influence offspring behaviour is wide, and includes emotional disturbances and events of a relatively subtle nature.
3. Offspring behaviour can be influenced during pregnancy by experiences undergone by the mother before mating or during infancy, and also by experiences undergone by the maternal grandparents.
4. The occurrence and quality of an effect on offspring behaviour depend on the interaction of a pre-natal influence with other variables, amongst which fetal genotype, stage of pregnancy, and post-natal experience are often particularly important.

2. The human studies: some problems of interpretation

Even the most careful of the studies on pre-natal influences on human behaviour have necessarily been relatively uncontrolled, with the result that there are bound to be many confusions and inconsistencies in the findings. There are thus many problems and uncertainties in any attempt to interpret the data in order to assess its implications for antenatal care, and for obstetric and paediatric practice. Nevertheless 'there is greater validity in drawing conclusions from studies of humans, despite their limitations, than in extrapolating from animal experiments without evidence from man' (Joffe, 1969).

The methodological problems involved in studies of pre-natal influences, both animal and human, have recently been discussed in detail (Joffe, 1969 a and b, Furchtgott, 1970). However, our present purpose is merely to draw attention to a few of the commoner and more important factors that influence the validity of the published reports. It is hoped, too, that this section will serve to provide some background to the research problems which may be of some practical assistance to obstetricians, paediatricians, and others in the maternity services who wish to interpret their own observations, or to design research on the behavioural implications of experiences during pregnancy.

It is frequently pointed out that it is because behaviour is a product of a very large number of variables which often interact significantly with each other, that sophisticated controls and analytic techniques are usually required in order to unravel any but the most major influences upon it. Many of the studies reviewed in the last section underlined the need to take account not only of the variables directly affecting a given individual, but also of those which affected his ancestors.

Whether an influence during pregnancy is likely to have an effect or not, together with the quality and direction of any effect, depends on the significance of its interactions with the rest of the variables significantly involved. These can include such groups of variables as genotype, ancestor experience, maternal uterine experience, maternal experience from birth through to pregnancy, as well as other maternal and fetal experiences during pregnancy and labour. It can also depend on its effect, together with that of all the other variables, on the mother's post-natal behaviour towards her child, or alternatively on the characteristics of any foster parent. Finally, and often crucially, it can depend on its interaction with the rest of the child's post-natal experience. The interactions likely to be significant will vary according to the pre-natal influence concerned.

Further, without appropriate controls, some of the effects of these groups of variables may easily be confounded with the effects of the pre-natal influence itself. In this respect, it is particularly important that the research design should be able to differentiate transmission of an influence to the child via the uterine environment from its transmission via the mother's milk or her post-natal behaviour. An additional complication is that an effect may not be apparent in the neonate, but show itself only at some later stage of development.

It is perhaps worth emphasizing at this point that many studies have indicated that both before and during pregnancy the behaviour of the father, or his absence, often forms a highly significant part of the maternal experiences in so far as these affect the fetus. Indeed, in some studies (e.g. Yerushalmy, 1962) the behaviour of the father during pregnancy is more strongly associated with the child's physiology or behaviour *at birth* than is the equivalent aspect of the mother's behaviour. In some cases it is possible that such effects are in part genetically mediated. In others, environmental mediation seems more likely, and is feasible in terms of physiological mechanisms.

To achieve some measure of control over the complex of variables, the animal experiments typically make use of elaborate rotating designs. Over several generations these systematically manipulate the strain of parents and foster parents, as well as their experiences at a number of points during their lives and pregnancies. To increase control, ova transplantation and caesarean delivery techniques have been contemplated (Joffe, 1969), but are hardly suitable for use in large-scale experiments.

Such degrees of control are neither possible nor desirable in studies of pre-natal influences on man and this means that only relatively powerful influences which operate on large numbers of people are likely to be detected, and even then not reliably. Although it is precisely these powerful influences which are likely to be of most general relevance in clinical practice, it should not be forgotten that the less easily identifiable influences are likely to contribute to at least some of the many differences in behaviour seen from birth onwards.

The human studies are typically not only naturalistic and non-experimental, but often the limited information available about patients leads to further difficulties through the use of impure variables. That is to say, the variables are often loosely defined, global, non-unitary, and overlap or operate through each other. For example, nutrition and social-class are often confounded in this way. Further, many variables affect some aspects of behaviour but not others, so that negative findings on whatever aspects of post-natal behaviour happen to have been observed and recorded may not be generalizable to other possibly more important aspects of behaviour.

Most of the published studies have been retrospective, and this creates additional difficulties for interpretation. Retrospective clinical studies tend to be overweighted with cases which have drawn attention to themselves through requiring treatment, and tend to miss other individuals in whom the interaction is such that the same pre-natal influence has had a milder effect, or no detectable effect at all. They are thus likely to overestimate the incidence of noxious effects from a given pre-natal influence, as happened in earlier investigations of rubella, for example (Tartakow, 1965). For similar reasons, positive effects of pre-natal influences are largely overlooked. The noxious effects tend to be further over-emphasized if, as often happens, the incidence of the effect in individuals who have not been exposed to the pre-natal influence concerned is not taken into account. To do this requires control groups, and raises further problems common to many uses of control groups in clinical studies. For example, some of the controls without histories of a particular influence may nevertheless have suffered an unrecorded exposure to it.

Retrospective studies can also suffer from the unreliability of retrospective diagnosis, and this is a particularly serious problem where data is derived from parents' recollections. The accuracy of parental memory for pregnancy events can be of such a low order by the time the child has reached the age of two years that this source of information has to be completely disregarded (Yarrow, 1963), and where the child has an evident problem the distortions are likely to be increased. Memories of the timing of events during pregnancy tend to be especially vulnerable, and in view of the demonstrated dependence of many effects on the precise stage of development when the influence occurs, this can be a major source of negative findings and misleading conclusions.

Some of these distortions can be avoided in prospective studies, which are gradually becoming more common, though they can introduce difficulties of their own. (Not least, problems of time and finance!) Interpretation of either type of study may be complicated by the problem of self-selected groups. For example, an apparent association between complications of pregnancy and lowered intelligence might be an artifact: both might be independent effects of inadequate nutrition. Alternatively, and more likely, lowered intelligence might result from nutritional deficiency both more or less directly, and indirectly via complications of pregnancy. Analysis of a random sample of pregnant mothers, rather than of a selected group of those suffering from complications of pregnancy, would increase confidence in any aetiological suggestions.

From the correlational and non-experimental nature of most of the human studies to be discussed in the next section, it follows that in any one investigation confident separation of pre-natal influences from genetic, pre-pregnancy, and post-natal factors is unlikely. However, when investigations using different techniques, and carried out in widely varying conditions, converge to implicate the same influences, greater confidence can be placed in the interpretations, and confidence will be further increased where animal studies implicate similar influences, or physiological investigations suggest likely mechanisms. Unravelling the interaction with post-natal factors is both particularly difficult, and also particularly important, in view of the immense demonstrated power of child-rearing practices to exacerbate, diminish, reverse, or otherwise modify the effects of pre-natal influences.

3. The human studies: some examples of the findings

One of the most comprehensive series of studies of pre-natal influences on man is that of Pasamanick and Knobloch and their associates (e.g. Pasamanick and Knobloch, 1966). They have put forward the concept of a 'continuum of reproductive causality': this emphasizes that, depending on its severity and interaction with other variables, an event during gestation may produce effects ranging from fetal or neonatal death to a graded series of sub-lethal conditions. These include neuropsychiatric disorders ranging from cerebral palsy, epilepsy, and mental deficiency to behaviour problems and reading difficulties. The concept of a continuum has three implications of immediate relevance. First, as an index of the relative toxicity of pre-natal influences, behaviour is likely to be more sensitive than morphology, although also more confounded. Second, milder doses of many of the influences already known to have fatal or severe morphological effects would be expected to have effects of considerable behavioural importance. And third, effects on behaviour are likely to be confounded with effects on mortality, morphology, and birth weight. The emphasis in this section is on behavioural effects uncomplicated by severe morphological effects. Although it will concentrate on effects for which considerable convergent evidence and feasible physiological mechanisms seem to exist, the many provisos implicit in section 2 are inevitably relevant throughout. For convenience, the studies will be grouped according to the major mechanisms likely to be involved, though interactions make such grouping largely arbitrary. The mechanisms themselves will be considered further in section 4. It is convenient to start with chemical influences, since besides their direct effects, they frequently mediate the more social influences.

CHEMICAL INFLUENCES

Nutrition. The doctrine of 'brain sparing' probably accounts, even more than the difficulties of data collection, for the lack of research until relatively recently on the influence of pre-natal nutrition on behaviour (Dobbing, 1967). However, although in the adult brain the quantity of all materials so far measured is unaffected even by starvation to death, during both pre-natal and post-natal brain development relatively mild nutritional deficits can have significant effects, and these can be particularly severe during 'vulnerable periods', such as E.C.A. 15–20 weeks, and E.C.A. 25 weeks till at least 60 weeks after birth (Dobbing and Sands, 1970). Inadequate diet during pregnancy may affect post-natal behaviour by a variety of routes: directly, by failing to meet the nutritional requirements of the fetus; or indirectly, by increasing the risk of maternal disease or complications of pregnancy; or before conception, by influencing the growth and development of the mother.

Although there are now a number of studies in progress, especially on protein deficiency, the main large-scale published report is that of Harrell, Woodyard, and Gates (1955), and this confined itself to an investigation of the effects of maternal vitamin supplementation on offspring pre-school intelligence. The vitamin supplement was administered to the mother during both late pregnancy and lactation, so that pre-natal and post-natal effects remain somewhat confounded. At 4 years of age the children of low-income mothers given the vitamin supplement achieved an average Terman-Merrill I.Q. 5·2 points higher than those of mothers given a placebo. Supplements had no significant effect on the children of higher-income mothers who were normally better nourished.

Less direct evidence is available from a number of sources. Many studies have shown strong associations between maternal nutrition and complications of pregnancy, and many others significant relationships between complications of pregnancy and various aspects of behaviour. Some of these studies will be discussed under 'Complications'. 'Light-for-dates' children show significant intellectual deficits in later life, and these may well be related to inadequate nutrition or placental insufficiency in late pregnancy (Dobbing, 1967). Likewise, in 27 pairs of monozygotic twins tested on W.I.S.C. between the ages of 5 and

15 years, significantly lower mean verbal and performance IQ scores were obtained by the lower birth weight twins (Willerman and Churchill, 1967). The effect was attributed to unequal sharing of inadequate nutrient supplies, resulting possibly from circulatory differences. Other investigators of twins have reported similar findings (Kaelber, 1969).

The scanty human data is strongly supported by the fast growing evidence from the rat. For example, although in the rat the most vulnerable period is after birth, a lipid-free diet during pregnancy results in severe impairment in offspring maze learning performance (Caldwell and Churchill, 1966). Equally severe impairments are found where maternal diets are deficient in protein or in vitamins, especially B-complex vitamins and folic acid (Timiras et al, 1968). Relatively mild nutritional deficiencies during the rat's vulnerable period, that is the three weeks from birth until weaning, lead to serious behavioural deficits, as well as parallel deficits in amount of myelin and number of neurones (Dobbing, 1967). These deficits are not rectified by abundant diet from weaning onwards, and persist through adult life. Neurochemical evidence on the importance of pre-natal and early post-natal nutrition in man has been obtained from studies of the brains of children who had died of malnutrition before the age of 12 months. These brains invariably show considerable reduction in cell number (D.N.A. index), and frequently the count is reduced to 40 per cent of normal (Wigglesworth, 1969). The deficit in cell number in those who survive is unremediable. Nevertheless, the long-term behavioural prognosis will depend on the interaction of the cell deficit with other variables, especially the early educational environment. Clearly, there is need for extensive further research on the influence of nutrition during pregnancy not only on human ability, but also on other aspects of behaviour, particularly attention and personality.

Oxygen. During their long series of investigations, Pasamanick and Knobloch (1966) found strong relationships between complications of pregnancy known to be accompanied by hypoxia and a range of syndromes, including cerebral palsy, epilepsy, mental retardation, reading difficulties, and behaviour problems. They proposed that degree of hypoxia was a major example of their 'continuum of reproductive causality'. Owing to the difficulties in collecting information on pre-natal hypoxia, most of the more direct human evidence comes from studies of perinatal hypoxia in full-term children, and of perinatal and post-natal hypoxia in prems. Typically, mild perinatal hypoxia tends to be associated with parallel degrees of poor motor co-ordination, reduced attention span, poor concentration and persistence, hyperactivity, impatience, irritability, and sometimes explosive temper tantrums. Mean IQ scores tend to be depressed, though to remain well within the 'normal' range, but the other characteristics tend to reduce the child's chances of fitting into the standard classroom situation, and sometimes lead to cumulative educational deficits. Which of these characteristics are primary and which secondary, the consequences either of attempts to cope with primary symptoms or of inappropriate rearing practices, remains to be clarified.

Typically, too, many of the symptoms tend to appear less pronounced as the child grows older. For example, one longitudinal study (Corah et al, 1965) found specific differences in intellectual functioning between mild hypoxics and normals up to the age of three years, with the hypoxics particularly poor on tests of concept formation. By eight years, however, the differences were less dramatic, but the hypoxics still showed significant attention difficulties and distractibility, as well as poor motor co-ordination. The association between hypoxia and cognitive impairment is further exemplified by a study which compared over 200 boys attending a clinic for reading difficulties with matched controls, and found a history of complications of pregnancy associated with hypoxia in 17 per cent of the poor readers, but in only 1·5 per cent of the controls (Kawi and Pasamanick, 1959). However, an association between hyperactivity and complications of pregnancy or perinatal hypoxia is by no means a universal finding (Stewart et al, 1966), and other variables are clearly importantly involved.

Hyperactivity is likely to be multi-determined, for example it is associated with other sources of brain damage, and both hyperactivity and complications of pregnancy can be independent consequences of other pre-natal factors, such as hormonal or emotional influences. Timing and degree of hypoxia, and hence brain areas tending to be most affected, are likely to be significant, and studies of relatively severe perinatal hypoxia in monkeys (Windle, 1968) reflect the association between human perinatal hypoxia and behavioural lethargy.

The studies of monkeys resuscitated after 8 minutes of perinatal asphyxiation support the human evidence of cognitive impairment (Windle, 1968). For example, severe memory deficits could still be demonstrated at the age of 10 years: delayed response performance failed after 5 seconds, whereas controls still succeeded at delays of more than 1 minute (Sechzer, 1969). Rats subjected to hypoxia early in gestation (gestational age 8 days) showed less activity and less emotionality than controls (Vierck et al, 1966), and pronounced impairments of maze and discrimination learning resulted from hypoxia at a gestational age 13–16 days (Meier et al, 1960).

The high incidence of prematurity and fetal and infant mortality in human societies at high altitudes, especially those living at over 10,000 feet (Grahn and Kratchman, 1963) suggests that the behavioural characteristics associated with mild pre-natal hypoxia would also be prevalent, but the existing data does not permit separation of the pre-natal, post-natal and cultural variables involved. Studies of attempts to improve fetal cerebral oxygenation and accelerate cerebral maturation through maternal ante-natal decompression remain at best inconclusive eight years after the initial reports from South Africa (Heyns et al, 1962). A well-controlled study which tested children on a developmental scale at 1, 4, and 9 months, and on Merrill-Palmer IQ at three years found no significant differences between the mean scores of decompression and control groups at any age (Liddicoat, 1968). Further, Liddicoat pointed out a number of possible sources of artifact in the original Heyns study. The findings of an E.E.G. investigation were equally negative (Murdoch, 1968). Thus, as far as intelligence scores are concerned, the value of decompression in uncomplicated pregnancies appears doubtful. However, its influence on other aspects of behaviour remains to be ascertained. And it has been suggested that its possible role in treating pre-eclampsia and ameliorating its consequences should be further investigated (B.M.J., 1968).

Hormones, sleep and emotion. Given adequate nutrition and oxygen, 'the most significant environmental factor to which the developing fetus is exposed is the influence of the endocrine system of its mother' (Woollam and Millen, 1960). Almost all chemico-hormonal changes in the maternal circulatory system, whether produced exogenously or endogenously, are likely to be reflected in the fetal circulation (Joffe, 1969). Despite this, little is yet known about the role of hormones on C.N.S. development before birth (Timiras et al, 1968). However, there are a large number of studies on the post-natal behavioural effects of hormonally mediated influences on the fetus. Only a few examples can be discussed here.

It has long been recognized that uncompensated maternal thyroid deficiency is associated in the child with a parallel degree of behavioural retardation, together with E.E.G. indications of malfunctioning, and reduction in size and amount of branching of cerebral cortical cells (Timiras et al, 1968).

The pre-natal role of androgens in man is unclear. In some mammals, for example rats, mice, and hamsters, secretion or administration of androgens at the critical stage of development leads to masculinization of the otherwise feminine hypothalamic activity patterns, and to corresponding effects on behaviour. These hypothalamic effects have not been found 'in rabbits, and probably not in monkeys, and so far, there is no evidence available that the human hypothalamus obeys the same type of androgenic organization' (Jost, 1970). Nevertheless, partial behavioural masculinization has been found in the female offspring of Rhesus monkeys to which testosterone was administered in the second quarter of gestation (Goy, 1968). And a careful investigation at the age of 10–12 years of 22 girls who had been exposed to androgens *in utero* indicated that they tended to be described by themselves and by others as tomboys, to engage in much rough-and-tumble play, and to prefer toys ordinarily associated with boys (Money and Ehrhardt, 1968). This has been described as 'a provocative study that will require replication and additional controls' (Hamburg, 1969).

The partial masculinization of the external genitalia of some girls exposed early in gestation to excessive amounts of some forms of progesterone is superficial, and, if corrected, apparently unaccompanied by effects on sexual behaviour. Of much greater practical importance is the influence of antenatal progesterone on intelligence. For example, one study (Dalton, 1968) followed up 90 children whose mothers had received a daily intramuscular administration of 50–300 mg of progesterone for the relief of toxaemic symptoms. As compared with matched controls, significantly more of the progesterone children were walking by 12 months, and at the age of 9–10 years they achieved significantly better grades in verbal reasoning, in English, arithmetic and academic subjects generally, and also in craftwork. The degree of developmental and intellectual advantage was related to total dosage, and was greatest when progesterone was received before the sixteenth week of gestation.

Further work is needed to ascertain the full significance of these findings. Meanwhile, the demonstration of a relationship between antenatal progesterone and intelligence has intriguing implications for the influence of maternal sleep habits on the fetus, and also for the use of the many drugs which modify the proportions of the different phases of sleep. During an extensive electrophysiological study of maternal sleep patterns at various stages of pregnancy (Petre-Quadens et al, 1969), an opportunity occurred to record fetal movements as well. In this subject (gestational age 33 weeks) it was found that fetal body movements were more frequent during maternal isolated-eye-movement sleep (40 per minute) and rapid-eye-movement sleep (21 per minute) than in the waking state (16 per minute), and were infrequent in the three stages of no-eye-movement sleep. During the eye-movement phase of sleep the mother and fetus are flooded with hormones, amongst which progesterone and growth hormone are of particular relevance here, especially as the proportion of maternal eye-movement sleep tends to increase throughout pregnancy. The fetal body-movement data provide further support for the proposal (Sterman and Jeannerod, 1967) that eye-movement sleep in the fetus occurs at the same time as it does in the mother, and suggest a common hormonal mediator. Further, similarities between the sleep-phase patterns of the newborn and of the mother after delivery suggest that the hormonal patterns set up by pre-natal maternal sleeping habits may influence the sleep of the child after birth, although there are other mechanisms which might also account for the relationship. The mechanisms through which hormones may exert such organizational influences on the developing C.N.S. will be briefly discussed in section 4.

The influence of catecholamines, especially adrenalin, in the maternal circulation has received extensive research. Joffe (1969) reviewed the many rat studies and, with provisos regarding interactions with other variables, summarized them thus: 'in general it appears that pre-natal administration of adrenalin increases emotionality . . . and probably decreases learning ability'. Here, attention will be confined to a few of the less direct human investigations, namely those concerning the influence of maternal emotional states during pregnancy. However, although the direct action of catecholamines plays an important part, many other mechanisms are likely to share responsibility for the correlations typically found with offspring behaviour. Amongst these other mechanisms adrenocortical and thyroid hormones, and hypothalamically mediated uterine influences figure prominently.

Careful recent investigations support the conclusions of the large number of less well controlled earlier studies, and the findings, which were reviewed in detail by Ferreira (1965) and Sontag (1966), can be summarized with fewer qualms than usual. The research has concentrated on the noxious influence of varying degrees of maternal emotional distress, ranging from mild tenseness and anxiety to the intense anxiety, grief or fear associated with illness or death in the family, severe matrimonial trouble, or housing problems. Other factors frequently involved include an unplanned pregnancy, an absent or disinterested husband, distress at interruption of career, and fears regarding childbirth and competence in child-rearing. Intense emotional upsets produce immediate and profound increases in fetal body movement, brief upsets leading to several hours of heightened irritability, and upsets lasting several weeks to hyperactivity throughout the entire period. In some extreme cases studied during the last trimester, ten-fold increases in body movements were observed (Sontag, 1941).

This fetal hyperactivity frequently persists after birth. Significant correlations have often been found between emotional distress during pregnancy and a group of offspring symptoms variously described as the 'difficult', 'colicky' or 'neurotic' child syndrome. Typically, from birth onward the infant shows increased irritability, restlessness, and fussiness, together with excessive crying. There is a high incidence of feeding difficulties, vomiting, frequent stools, and other signs of gastro-intestinal dysfunction. Duration of sleep tends to be reduced, whereas reactivity to sound is enhanced, being characterized by violent startle responses and loud crying. The long-term prognosis depends importantly on the interaction with post-natal experience, and particularly on parental reactions to coping with a 'difficult' child. Frequently, however, by the age of 2–3 years a marked shyness and lack of confidence are apparent, and exemplified by poor initiative, apprehensiveness in social contacts, and reluctance to join in play.

Correlations between maternal emotional distress and complications of pregnancy have been found in many investigations, and have been reviewed by Davids (1968) and McDonald (1968). Their interpretation raises many problems. Nevertheless, it seems that in some cases maternal emotions are indeed associated with complications, and can lead to the behavioural after-effects of complications which will be discussed later in this section. Anxiety is the emotion typically involved, and the complications associated with it range from hyperemesis and anomalous presentation to low birth weight, pre-eclampsia, habitual abortion, and infant mortality.

Maternal emotions can influence the fetus by routes other than direct hormonal ones. For example, fear-evoking stimuli produce great increases in uterine motility (Kelly, 1962). The absorption and retention of nutrients, particularly of calcium, phosphorus, and nitrogen, is seriously reduced during severe emotional distress. Further, significant relationships have been claimed between emotional stress before or during conception and such variables as sex ratio (Schuster and Schuster) and the incidence of Down's syndrome (Drillien and Wilkinson, 1964).

After his detailed and rigorously critical review of the many animal studies, Joffe (1969) was able to state: 'The conclusive demonstration in animal experiments that maternal emotional stress affects offspring behaviour means that the general proposition of the human studies is not implausible: it is quite likely that a human mother's emotional state during pregnancy will affect her child's behaviour.' The human investigations summarized here appear to justify this extrapolation, and emphasize the scope for further work, particularly on the less distressing emotions.

Maternal metabolism, age, and disease. Despite the massive literature on cases where morphological anomalies are present, there are very few published studies of behavioural effects of these variables where morphology is absent. Nevertheless, correlations have been shown between maternal B.M.R. and fetal body movements, and particularly close ones between changes in maternal B.M.R. and fetal activity in late pregnancy (Richards et al, 1938). An example of the influence of a maternal metabolic anomaly is provided by a study of 69 non-P.K.U. children of P.K.U. mothers. All but one showed serious motor and IQ impairment (Castells et al, 1968). The commonly found increasing incidence of complications of pregnancy and mental retardation in the offspring of mothers under 23 and over 35 seems to be related in part to the waxing and waning of the ability of the total maternal system to provide an optimum environment for fetal development. If the Pasamanick and Knobloch continuum is to be upheld, it would be expected that behavioural effects would be detectable even in the absence of severe complications or retardation. More work is required on the purely behavioural effects of the milder cases of maternal conditions which are likely to curtail the fetal oxygen supply, for example anaemia, hypertension, diabetes, and respiratory diseases.

In view of the possibly misleading impression created by earlier retrospective studies of virus diseases of the rubella type, it is perhaps worth drawing attention to Sheridan's (1964) prospective study of rubella in early pregnancy. Over 30 per cent of the offspring showed morphological abnormalities but at 8–11 years the mean IQ of the whole group was 106, with a range of 63–160, in other words very similar to the distribution for 'normal' children. Sheridan concluded that there was little evidence of intellectual impairment, or of emotional problems.

Drugs and smoking. Once again, the animal studies are suggestive. They show clearly that, depending on genotype, dosage, and stage of pregnancy when administered, a wide variety of common pharmacological agents can produce effects on offspring behaviour in the absence of overt morphological anomalies (Joffe, 1969). The human studies have tended to concentrate on medication during labour, and have shown even light sedation to be associated with depression of attention, feeding, and sucking behaviour for up to 8 days after birth (e.g. Stechler, 1964; Kron et al, 1966). Recent data (Richards, 1969) indicates an urgent need for research on the effects on offspring behaviour of aspirin during pregnancy.

Studies on the behavioural effects of smoking during pregnancy are lacking. However, the regularly found association (e.g. Butler, 1969) between smoking and a higher incidence of low birth weight, complications of pregnancy, and fetal mortality suggests that behavioural effects might well be found (see note on page 201). Support comes from the known properties of the constituents of tobacco smoke, particularly their vasoconstrictive and oxygen-competitive effects, and from the sudden and pronounced changes in fetal heart rate that can occur in response to the smoking of a single cigarette (Sontag and Wallace, 1935).

Season of birth. There is no lack of human data in this area. In the northern hemisphere there appears to be a higher incidence of complications of pregnancy, infant mortality and mental retardation in children born in January, February, and March (e.g. Pasamanick and Knobloch, 1966), and in a recent analysis of 23,000 mental patients the same trend was found for schizophrenia (Hare and Price, 1969). Not only is there a higher incidence of retardation (IQ<70) among winter-born children, but there are a number of reports of a seasonal trend in mean IQ within retardate groups, it being lowest for winter births (e.g. Orme, 1965; Berghund, 1967). Conflict and controversy characterizes the current picture presented by the large number of studies of the relationship with IQ and school achievement in 'normal' children. Nevertheless, despite a considerable number of discordant findings and confounding with many other variables, especially school organization and time-of-entry effects, the overall trend if anything seems again to be unfavourable to winter-born children.

Many attempts have been made to explain these seasonal effects, but that of Pasamanick and Knobloch (1966) seems best supported by evidence. They suggested a relationship with mild dietary deficiencies during the third month of gestation when the cortex is being organized, and produced evidence of a significant decrease in food intake, particularly calorie and protein intake, during hot weather (at least in U.S. urban families). Their data also shows a slightly higher incidence of retardate births in the winters following hot summers than those following cool ones. If they are right, the effects can presumably be eliminated by attention to diet, but the matter remains controversial.

PHYSICAL INFLUENCES

Radiation. The influence of intrauterine radiation on human behaviour seems to have been little studied except when associated with morphological effects. In the rat, however, a wide range of behaviour has been shown to be affected without overt morphological signs. The range includes motor performance, emotionality, activity level, learning ability, and mating behaviour (Joffe, 1969).

MECHANICAL AND SENSORY INFLUENCES

Pressure, touch, and movement. Mechanical stimulation from maternal uterine, heart, respiratory, and gross bodily movements has long-term significance for the fetus (e.g. Sontag, 1966). Such stimulation is likely to influence developmental rate and arousal level. For example, incubator prems who were mechanically rocked at 12 excursions per minute for half-an-hour twice daily were more relaxed and showed more spontaneous smiling while being rocked. They also gained weight faster than controls, which included 9 identical co-twins (Freedman, 1969). The reflex movements of the fetus in response to touch, which appear at 7 weeks of gestational age, have been described in detail (e.g. Humphrey, 1964) and are likely to play an important part in morphological as well as behavioural development. Fetal mouth-opening reflexes, for example, appear to be essential for normal palate formation, and anomalies of development are associated with drugs and other influences which reduce such activity (Humphrey, 1969a). Tactile and kinesthetic self-stimulation, for example the thumb-sucking behaviour recorded in the second trimester, may be involved in the maintenance of an activity level adequate for good pre-natal muscular development.

Position. The walking and crawling reflexes appear to help the fetus to move around the uterus until it gets into the right position for a vertex presentation. The posture and position of the infant for weeks after birth tend to vary according to the intrauterine position in the last weeks before birth. This is found, for example, in babies born in breech or face presentation, and they also show anomalous and reversed reflexes (Prechtl, 1969), as well as atypical E.E.G.s (Ellingson, 1967). Significant relationships have been reported between head position at birth and the IQ of school-age children. Among 212 subjects for whom the necessary data were available, verbal scores were significantly lower than performance scores in those whose delivery had been occiput-right. No significant differences were found between verbal and performance scores for occiput-left deliveries. This possibly suggests that the left hemisphere, normally the 'speech' hemisphere, is more vulnerable during occiput-right deliveries (Churchill et al, 1968).

Sound. Fetal responses to sound during the last trimester *in utero* are well documented, and occur independently of maternal mediation (e.g. Dwornicka et al, 1964). A sudden loud sound, such as a doorbell, produces an immediate acceleration of fetal heart rate, and usually a startle reflex followed by violent kicking and body movement. It has been suggested (Sontag, 1966) that exposure to spasmodic loud noise for relatively prolonged periods during pregnancy may lead to chronic fetal hyperactivity, similar to that associated with maternal emotional distress. Further, a number of clinical reports indicate a relation between noisy environments during pregnancy and the colicky or hyperactive child syndrome. This relation is supported by the finding that emotionality is increased in rats subjected *in utero* to the frequent sounding of a buzzer (Morra, 1965). Other human studies, to be discussed in section 4, suggest that neonatal sensory preferences, including auditory and rhythmic ones, are related to sensory experiences *in utero*.

COMPLICATIONS

On average the behavioural effects of complications of pregnancy and delivery, multiple pregnancy and low birth weight appear to be confounded with and often swamped by the lifestyle and child-rearing variables usually unhappily classified as social-class variables. Nevertheless, the results of investigations that have taken pains to achieve a measure of separation of some of the factors involved suggest that some complications *per se* can sometimes have influences of practical importance.

Complications of pregnancy. Most of the available studies have suffered through being retrospective and from the difficulties of providing valid controls. Further, many of them have tended to group a variety of very different conditions together as 'complications', and so consistently significant results are hardly to be expected, and indeed not found. For example, in the area of 'disturbed behaviour' at school, an early investigation of 2,000 cases amongst schoolchildren in Baltimore found a higher incidence of complications, especially toxaemia (Pasamanick et al, 1956), and similar results were obtained in a Scottish study (Drillien, 1963). On the other hand, another Scottish investigation of 100 cases came up with negative findings (Wolff, 1967). The position appears similar for psychiatric disorders, for example childhood schizophrenia, although some studies have found 'conclusive evidence of more reproductive complications' (Taft and Goldfarb, 1964). Conflicting results also characterize surveys of the influence on IQ. A comprehensive early study (Pasamanick and Lilienfeld, 1955; Kawi and Pasamanick, 1959) found a significantly greater incidence of complications in retardates and in children with reading difficulties than in matched controls. But a representative survey of all children born in Birmingham from 1950–65 resulted in negative findings (Barker, 1966).

It thus appears that any behavioural influence of complications of pregnancy is often so dependent on interactions with other factors that a realistic assessment of its overall importance will have to await the outcome of some of the more controlled large-scale prospective studies now in progress.

Birth weight and length of gestation

Child-rearing and socio-economic variables also interact strongly with the factors associated with low birth weight (see the discussion of 'Social Class' later in this section). However, significant birth weight effects appear to remain after these variables have been taken into consideration. For example, in a survey of 1,000 children aged 4 years, it was found that in the prems level of intelligence was directly related to degree of prematurity (Drillien and Ellis, 1964). A similar relationship was demonstrated in a longitudinal study to the age of 13 years of over 400 children with birth weight of under 2,500 g. Compared with matched full-term controls, they showed as a group intellectual impairments which increased as a function of decreasing birth weight, although many individual children appeared unaffected. With social class and maternal practices apparently taken into account, significant deficits could still be detected in a wide range of tests of motor ability, intelligence, speech, reading, and school achievement. The impairments were associated with indications of neurological defect (Wiener, 1968). The data for identical twins already discussed under 'Nutrition' is consistent with this picture: the mean IQ score for the lighter children in each pair was significantly lower than that for the heavier ones. Intriguingly, no significant differences were found for a group of fraternal twins (Churchill, 1965).

The low birth weight effect may sometimes be related in part to a period of under-stimulation in an incubator, or to overprotection and less cognitive pushing by parents (e.g. Caplan et al, 1963; Salk, 1968). High birth weight is also associated with intellectual impairment. For example, children of birth weight over 4,200 g showed more than twice the normal incidence of IQ under 80 (Babson et al).

In general, the birth weight data appear to reflect the retarded growth and neurological anomalies associated with the chemical influences already discussed. However, though birth weight has the advantage of being an easily collected statistic, it is a crude index of developmental level or neurological integrity, and for fuller study of the behavioural implications of growth *in utero*, more sophisticated measures are necessary, such as those provided by the E.E.G.

SOCIAL INFLUENCES

Highly significant interactions with 'social' variables have been found in a majority of the surveys of pre-natal influences on behaviour. Despite their importance, there is space here for no more than a few examples and comments.

The Father. 'Marital adjustment', 'absent father', and 'illegitimacy' often loom large among the factors associated with maternal emotional stress, and the 'colicky child' syndrome that often results (e.g. Tupper and Weil, 1962). More controlled studies of paternal influences are required, particularly in the light of such intriguing findings as those of Yerushalmy (1962), whose data indicated that children's birth weight was more closely associated with the smoking habits of their fathers than with those of their mothers.

Population density. Problems of pregnancy and child behaviour figure prominently among the many disorders and diseases which public health records for large cities typically show to increase in frequency as a function of population density. Although many other factors clearly play major roles, the animal and physiological data suggest that direct and indirect effects of population density *per se* may be of importance. Many rodent studies, for example, have shown that mothers overcrowded during pregnancy produce pups showing impaired learning ability, increased emotionality, and other behaviour disturbances (e.g. Keeley, 1962).

Social class. The various crude indices of 'socio-economic status' often reflect in part such social variables as 'way-of-life', mode of child-rearing and attitude to education as well as factors like feeding habits, food availability and quality of obstetric care. A strong interaction with obstetric variables affecting behaviour might thus be expected, and is certainly found. The very pronounced association of socio-economic status with incidence of obstetric problems (e.g. Butler, 1969) is paralleled by its equally pronounced association with level of intelligence and achievement (Vernon, 1969).

Child-rearing practices and the educational background of the home play a highly significant part in the development of intelligence, and this is clearly demonstrated in the many studies reviewed by Vernon. For example, Douglas (1964) compared 650 prems with full-term controls on tests of intelligence and school achievement. On average, the prems scored lower when tested at both 8 and 11 years. But prems from good homes scored as well as full-term children from good homes; prems from poor homes scored lower than both full-term and prem children from good homes; and, most revealingly, the prems from good homes scored higher than the full-term children from poor homes. Good or poor homes were defined in terms of the socio-economic status of both parents, mother's child-care rating and parental interest in the educational progress of the child. Further, in the prem group the number of children from poor homes was three times the number from good homes.

Many other surveys (e.g. Robinson and Robinson, 1964) support the conclusion that in many populations the interactions are typically such that social class is often much more important than birth weight in determining the long-term intellectual prognosis, and the position appears similar for mild complications of pregnancy (Douglas, 1964). In other words, a number of pre-natal factors which vary according to social-class, particularly diet and ante-natal care, have important behavioural effects, which can be either greatly exacerbated or greatly ameliorated by post-natal factors, such as diet in the first year or so and child-rearing practices, which also vary according to social class.

In the absence of the powerful educational influences that can break the vicious circle, these effects can be self-perpetuating across generations. Sub-optimal conditions, either dietary or social, during pre-natal and post-natal development can produce girls whose impaired functional and behavioural efficiency renders them less able to provide their own children with favourable pre-natal and post-natal environments. Such mechanisms could account for some of the 'granny' and 'grandpa' effects that have been observed. For example,

Drillien (1957) found the incidence of prematurity to be more highly correlated with the socio-economic status of the maternal grandfather than with that of the father, and suggested the link was produced through the mother's nutritional history and childhood health. A behavioural example is provided by the first Perinatal Mortality Survey. A significant correlation was found between reading difficulties at the age of 7 years, and the mother's social environment before she started her schooling. Throughout development over many generations chemical and cultural factors combine to influence the behaviour mediated by the 'normal' human brain.

4. Some mechanisms

Discussion of the mechanisms underlying pre-natal influences on human behaviour is perhaps premature. Most of the mechanisms which will be mentioned have been demonstrated in physiological preparations, but some, though plausible, have hypothetical status only. How far they actually apply *in utero* is often not yet known.

During much of the development of the brain, structure and function mutually influence each other, and the structural substrates of later behaviour are thus often modified by earlier behaviour and experience. 'In a material sense much of the brain is made while its functioning is in progress. . . . Electrical activity begins in the brain before the greater part of its substance has been assembled. From this point, material growth of the brain progresses while it is receiving impulses from the rest of the body and the environment in which that body exists' (McIlwain, 1966).

CHEMICAL VULNERABILITY

The vulnerability of the brain to nutritional deficiencies seems to be greatest during the two major growth spurts, or periods of rapid cell multiplication, when it is likely that even comparatively mild restrictions can produce permanent cell deficits. Restrictions from the fifteenth to twentieth weeks of conceptual age, when rapid neuroblast proliferation is likely to be occurring, may lead to reduction in the number of neurones formed. Malnutrition between 25 weeks of conceptual age and the second year of life, the period of active glial division, probably leads to an ultimate deficit in glial cells and myelination (Dobbing and Sands, 1970).

Windle (1969) has described the cell losses in various parts of the brains of monkeys subjected to short periods of perinatal hypoxia. He emphasizes that perinatal asphyxia which lasts long enough to require resuscitation inevitably produces permanent damage. Further, the initial cell losses can lead to further losses months after birth. For example, destruction of thalamic cells leads to the gradual atrophy and disappearance of the cortical neurones to which they radiate.

METABOLIC ADAPTATION AND BIOCHEMICAL INDIVIDUALITY

McIlwain (1970) has drawn attention to the influence of environmental factors on the metabolic adaptation of the brain during its development. Not only may enzyme induction 'play a part in the initial growth of the brain by favouring particular synaptic connections in a manner related to sensory input', but altered sensory input can lead via alterations in cerebral functioning to persisting changes in the enzyme composition of the brain. Since hormones at a suitable time can act as a genetic switch in deciding a route of development, much differentiation during development is irreversible. Perinatal metabolic adaptations in the rat, due to thyroxin deficiency for example, have been shown to last a lifetime. Even the availability of an amino acid at a critical time can permanently alter the expression of genetic potential, and possibly lead to cumulative developmental misprogramming and dysfunction. In other words, 'the multiplicity of enzymatically based adaptations' of which the brain is capable form a system likely to respond with great sensitivity throughout its development to environmental influences.

Environmentally produced adaptations of this sort may play

a part, together with genetic influences, in bringing about the pronounced 'biochemical individuality' found by Williams (1956). There have been frequent demonstrations of associations between biochemical differences and various aspects of intellectual and emotional behaviour. For example, the correlations found between urinary constituents and intellectual abilities in school children and university students (King et al, 1961; Sanders et al, 1960).

STIMULATION LEVEL

Since the work of Krech et al (1960), there have been extensive studies of the influence of sensory stimulation on the chemical composition of the developing brain, and on the rate of growth of both brain and body. For example, level of stimulation of the infant rat is associated with rate of increase in neuroglial cells (Timiras et al, 1968).

Stimulation level may also have long-term behavioural effects through endocrine mechanisms. Levine and Mullins (1966) have proposed that control of some hormonal functions in adult organisms is partially accomplished by means of a 'hormonostat', or hormone feedback mechanism, whose range and sensitivity is determined by hormonal levels during development. These, in turn, vary according to the level of stimulation to which the developing organism is exposed. It has been suggested (Petre-Quadens et al, 1969) that inappropriate stimulation of the brain-endocrine feedback mechanisms during intrauterine life may lead to some forms of intellectual impairment.

Some of the functions of the autonomic nervous system may also be organized or 'tuned' by stimulation levels *in utero*. Electrocardiographic studies have demonstrated large individual differences in fetal autonomic reactivity, as well as correlations between fetal and maternal patterns of reactivity: 'labile' mothers had the most active fetuses in terms of both cardiac responses and body movement (Sontag, 1966). Genetic influences may be partly responsible for these correlations.

Autonomic reactivity is strongly related to a number of personality variables.

LEARNING *in utero*

Controversy still reigns over the possibility of intrauterine learning, though much of it has arisen over differences of definition. Despite the controversy there has been remarkably little direct research, and there are few clear-cut findings. The 'classical' study is that of Spelt (1948) who used Pavlovian conditioning procedures with a group of fetuses in their last trimester *in utero*. He was able to set up a body movement response to a signal in the form of a mild vibration. Although a careful investigation, complete control of various sources of artifact was inevitably not obtained, and criticism and scepticism have been frequent. Neonatal conditioning is dependent on the 'state' of the child (see Prechtl, 1969). It is unlikely that the earlier attempts at fetal conditioning would have succeeded without taking into account recent findings on 'state', and this may be a reason for the negative results, though hardly for Spelt's positive ones. The use of recently developed techniques should soon produce a more conclusive picture.

However, there is more to learning than conditioning, which constitutes a rather special case. Many workers consider that some of the correlations found between intrauterine and postnatal characteristics indicate a form of learning. It has been suggested, for example, that the relationship between intrauterine position and neonatal posture implies learning (e.g. Bronson, 1969). Similarly, the sensory preferences shown by neonates in 'cafeteria' experiments (see Lipsitt, 1969), have led to the speculation that sensory expectations or 'adaptation levels' may be acquired *in utero*, and that distress and crying occur when current experience fails to match these learned expectations. An example is provided by the reduction in crying and activity in neonates exposed to rhythmic stimulation such as sound or rocking at a frequency close to that of the maternal heart beat (Salk, 1962; Ambrose, 1969). Additional evidence comes from animal experiments (Grier et al, 1967).

Metabolic adaptation and endocrine and autonomic tuning can all be regarded as mechanisms of learning. And J. Z. Young's concept of 'tissue memory' clearly applies to the developing fetus. The role of the cortex is uncertain, though the E.E.G. studies discussed in the Introduction suggest it could be partly functional. Possibly the question 'Does learning occur *in utero?*' is an unfortunate one. It might be less confusing to ask 'Do intrauterine events influence later behaviour?', and here the answer is more straightforward.

5. Some practical implications

At the end of his examination of the methodological status of the human research, Joffe (1969) concluded: 'The human studies provide sufficient evidence to enable preventive pre-natal action to be initiated with regard to a variety of pregnancy and childhood disorders without waiting for the methodological issues to be unravelled precisely – though the action may be more effective when they are.' The action to be taken is usually clearly implicit in the findings themselves. This section looks at a few studies which throw further light on some of the implications for antenatal and child care.

ANTENATAL CARE

Amount of antenatal care often turns out to be the most important difference between the mothers of full-term and premature children living in the same underprivileged area (Freedman, 1962). It is likely to have an even greater effect on the initial behaviour of the child, and through this on long-term development.

Dietary recommendations seem even more important than previously recognized. The behavioural findings strongly support the suggestion that the obstetric practice in some countries of keeping weight gain during pregnancy to a minimum should be modified. Better behavioural development during the first year, as well as higher birth weight and decreased prematurity and infant mortality, are found where higher maternal weight gain is encouraged (Singer et al, 1968). Restriction of weight gain to as little as 10–14 lb, as recently practised in the U.S., seems particularly associated with increased problems. It is likely that, in addition to the obstetric complications that often accompany them, reductions in weight gain from about the thirty-fourth week onwards have important implications for behaviour.

The emotional and social aspects of maternity pose far less tractable problems. Many of the social habits that influence behaviour pre-natally are deeply ingrained and highly resistant to change. Nevertheless, knowledge of the behavioural implications can be of assistance in the planning of pregnancies. Particularly, the repercussions of the physical and emotional immaturity of the mother, unwanted pregnancies, the father's behaviour, marital and other emotional discord, accommodation problems, fatigue and noise, and distress at interrupting employment (Ferreira, 1965). A formidable list! A number of practitioners have claimed considerable success, including a reduction in incidence of obstetric complications, from treating emotional problems during pregnancy through psychotherapy (Tupper and Weil, 1962; Knobel, 1967).

PREDICTION OF POST-NATAL BEHAVIOUR FROM FETAL BEHAVIOUR

Maternal attitudes during pregnancy can be useful predictors of offspring behaviour (Doty, 1967). But more direct predictions can be made by assessing fetal behaviour itself. Earlier studies which used maternal reports of fetal activity for this purpose, and found high correlations with behavioural development at 6 and 12 months of age, were open to various forms of artifact (Richards and Newberry, 1938; Walters, 1965). However, in some circumstances the reliability of maternal reports can be high. For example, mothers of fraternal twins sometimes report that one moves much more than the other before birth, and post-natally one twin turns out to be active and the other lethargic (Humphrey, 1969). Whether these differences reflect genotype or mechanical or circulatory differences at some stage of development is unclear.

Objective measures of fetal activity were used in the Fels Longitudinal studies (Sontag, 1966). Sizable correlations were found between the variability of fetal heart rate and the variability of resting heart rate even at the age of 20 years. There was a definite tendency for fetal cardiac labiles to become adult labiles, and stabiles showed a similar consistency over time. This has important implications for behaviour, in view of the strong association between cardiac responsivity and personality characteristics. For example, labiles tend to be more imaginative and emotional.

In general, there is a strong relationship between fetal activity level and infant behaviour characteristics. Further, individual differences in personality apparent in the first weeks of life tend to persist. In a highly controlled longitudinal study up to the age of 14 years (Thomas et al, 1970), cluster analysis identified three main personality patterns, classified as 'easy children', 'difficult children', and 'children slow to warm up'. As neonates the 'difficult children' showed all the characteristics of the 'colicky child syndrome', discussed in section 3, and associated with emotional distress during pregnancy. Seventy per cent of these 'difficult children' developed severe behaviour problems, whereas only eighteen per cent of the 'easy children' did so. The study followed the development of personality as it was gradually shaped by the constant interplay of physiological characteristics and environment.

Pre-natal influences clearly form a significant part of that environment. The child is born with an individuality which is a product of the interaction of genotype and pre-natal environment. The future development of the child then depends on matching rearing practices to his particular characteristics. The same practices have different consequences, depending on the characteristics of the particular infant, and this needs to be taken into account when advice is given on weaning, toilet training, handling, or upbringing in general. This process is cumulative, and the long-term prognosis depends on the continual adjustment of the rearing and educational treatment of the child to match the existing mix. Provided damage to the brain is not too severe, the influence of an effective upbringing of this sort can often swamp even serious obstetric problems. Where the post-natal environment is not so favourable, handicaps developed *in utero* may be exacerbated. To twist the meaning of an old saying, 'Birth is much, but breeding more'.

N.B.—Since this was written, the suggestion has been confirmed. In the follow-up of the Perinatal Mortality Survey (1958 cohort) at seven years, Southgate reading scores of children whose mothers had smoked during pregnancy were significantly lower than those of controls, and this effect remained significant even with children of low birth weight partialled out. (Butler, Personal Communication.)

References

ADER, R., and DEITCHMAN, R. (1970). 'Effect of pre-natal maternal handling on the maturation of rhythmic processes', *J. comp. physiol. Psychol.*, **71**(**3**), 492.

AMBROSE, A. (1969). Ed. *Stimulation in Early Infancy*, 103–4 (London and New York: Academic Press).

BABSON, S. G., HENDERSON, N. B., and CLARK, W. M. 'Pre-school intelligence of oversized newborns', *Proc. 77th Annual Conv. APA*, **4** (Pt. 1), 267.

BARKER, D. J. P. (1966). 'Low intelligence and obstetric complications', *Br. J. prev. soc. Med.*, **20**, 15.

BERGHUND, G. W. (1967). 'Intelligence and season of birth', *Br. J. Psychol.*, **58**(**1–2**), 147.

BERGSTROM, R. M. (1969). 'Electrical parameters of the brain during ontogeny', ed. Robinson, R. J. *Brain and Early Behaviour*, 15 (London and New York: Academic Press).

BRIT. MED. J. (1964). **1**, 1064. 'Pre-natal shaping of behaviour.'

—— (1968). **2**, 317. 'Abdominal decompression during pregnancy.'

BRONSON, G. (1969). In ed. Robinson, R. J., *Brain and Early Behaviour*, 76 (London and New York: Academic Press).

BUTLER, N. (1969). 'Perinatal problems.' Second Report, Perinatal mortality Survey (Edinburgh and London: E. and S. Livingstone).

CALDWELL, D. F., and CHURCHILL, J. A. (1966). 'Learning impairment in rats administered lipid-free diet during pregnancy', *Psychol. Reports*, **19**(**1**), 99.

CAPLAN, H., BIBACE, R., and RABINOVITCH, M. S. (1963). 'Paranatal stress, cognitive organization and ego function', *J. Child Psychiat.*, **2**, 434.

CASTELLS, S., and BRANDT, I. K. (1968). 'Phenylketonuria: evaluation of therapy and verification of diagnosis', *J. Pediat.*, **72**, 34.

CHURCHILL, J. A., WILLERMAN, L., GRISELL, J., and AYERS, M. A. (1968). 'Effect of head position at birth on WISC verbal and performance IQ', *Psychol. Reports*, **23**(**2**), 495.

CORAH, N. L., ANTHONY, E. J., PAINTER, P., STERN, J. A., and THURSTON, D. (1965). 'Effects of perinatal anoxia after 7 years', *Psychol. Monogr.*, **79**, 1.

DALTON, K. (1968). 'Antenatal progesterone and intelligence', *Br. J. Psychiat.*, **114**, 1377.

DAVIDS, A. (1968). 'A research design for studying maternal emotionality before childbirth and after social interaction with the child', *Merrill-Palmer Quart.*, **14**(**4**), 344.

DENENBERG, V. H. (1969). 'Experimental programming of life histories in the rat', ed. Ambrose, A. *Stimulation in early Infancy*, 21, (London and New York: Academic Press).

——, and ROSENBERG, K. M. (1967). 'Nongenetic transmission of information', *Nature*, **216**, 549.

—— —— (1968). 'Effects of maternal and environmental variables upon open-field behaviour', *Devel. Psychobiol.*, **1**(**2**), 93.

——, and WHIMBEY, A. E. (1963). 'Behaviour of adult rats is modified by experiences their mothers had as infants', *Science*, **142**, 1192.

DOBBING, J. (1967). 'Growth of the brain', *Sci. J.*, **3**, **5**, 81.

——, and SANDS, J. (1970). 'Timing of neuroblast multiplication in developing human brain', *Nature*, **226**, 639.

DOTY, B. A. (1967). 'Relationships among attitudes in pregnancy and other maternal characteristics', *J. Genetic Psychol.*, **111**(**2**), 203.

DOUGLAS, J. W. B. (1964). *The Home and the School* (London: McGibbon and Kee).

DRILLIEN, C. M. (1957). 'Social and economic factors affecting the incidence of premature birth', *J. Obst. Gynec. Br. Commonw.*, **64**, 161.

—— (1963). 'Obstetric hazard, mental retardation and behaviour disturbances in primary school', *Devel. Med. child Neurol.*, **5**(**1**), 3.

——, and ELLIS, R. W. B. (1964). *The Growth and Development of the Prematurely Born Infant* (Baltimore: Williams and Wilkins).

——, and WILKINSON, E. M. (1964). 'Emotional stress and mongoloid births', *Devl. Med. Child Neurol.*, **6**, 140.

DWORNICKA, B., JASLENSKA, A., SMOLARZ, W., and WAWRYK, R. (1964). 'Attempt of determining fetal reaction to acoustic stimulation', *Acta Oto-Laryngologica*, **57**, 571.

ELLINGSON, R. J. (1967). 'Brain electrical activity in infants', eds. Lipsitt, L. P., and Spiker, C. C. *Advances in Child Development and Behaviour*, Vol. 3 (London and New York: Academic Press).

FERREIRA, A. J. (1965). 'Emotional factors in pre-natal environment: a review', *J. nerv. ment. Dis.*, **141**, **1**, 108.

FRASER, F. C. (1964). 'Experimental teratogenesis in relation to congenital malformations in man', ed. Fishbein, M. *Second International Conference on Congenital Malformations*, 277 (New York: International Medical Congress).

FREEDMAN, A. M. (1962). 'Long range anterospective study of premature infants', *World Mental Health*, **14**(**1**), 9.

FREEDMAN, D. G. (1969). In ed. Ambrose, A. *Stimulation in Early Infancy*, 102 (London and New York: Academic Press).

FURCHTGOTT, E. (1970). 'Behaviour begins before birth', *Contemp. Psychol.*, **15**, **5**, 326.

GOY, R. W. (1969). In ed. Michael, R. *Endocrinology and Human Behaviour*, 12 (London: Oxford University Press).

GRAHN, D., and KRATCHMAN, J. (1963). 'Variation in neonatal death rate in U.S., and possible relations to environment, radiation, geology and altitude'. *Amer. J. Hum. Gen.*, **15**, 329.

GRIER, J. B., COUNTER, S. A., and SHEARER, W. M. (1967). 'Pre-natal auditory imprinting in chicks', *Science*, **155**(**3770**), 1692.

HAMBURG, D. A. (1969). 'A combined biological and psychosocial approach to the study of behavioural development', ed. Ambrose, A. *Stimulation in Early Infancy*, 269 (London and New York: Academic Press).

HARE, E. H., and PRICE, J. S. (1969). 'Mental disorder and season of birth', *Br. J. Psychiat.*, **115**(**522**), 533.

HARRELL, R. F., WOODYARD, E., and GATES, A. J. (1955). *The Effects of Mothers' Diets on the Intelligence of Offspring* (New York: Teacher's College, Columbia University).

HEYNS, O. S., SAMSON, J. M., and ROBERTS, W. A. B. (1962). 'An analysis of infants whose mothers had decompression during pregnancy', *Med. Proc.*, **8**, 307.

HRBEK, A., KARLBERG and OLSSON (1970). 'Assessment of maturity of premature children by variations in evoked responses', Paper presented at Second European Congress of Perinatal Medicine, London, April 1970.

HUMPHREY, T. (1964). 'Some correlations between the appearance of human fetal reflexes and the development of the nervous system', *Prog. Brain Res.*, **4**, 93.

—— (1969a). 'The relation between human fetal mouth opening reflexes and closure of the palate', *Am. J. Anat.*, **125**, 317.

—— (1969b). 'Post-natal repetition of human prenatal activity sequences' ed. Robinson, R. J. *Brain and Early Behaviour*, 43 (London and New York: Academic Press).

JOFFE, J. M. (1969). *Prenatal Determinants of Behaviour* (Oxford: Pergamon Press).

JOST, A. D. (1970). 'Development of sexual characteristics', *Sci. J.*, **6**(**6**), 67.

KAELBER, C. T. et al (1969). 'Influence of intrauterine relations on intelligence of twins', *New Engl. J. Med.*, **280**, 1030.

KAWI, A. A., and PASAMANICK, B. (1959). 'Pre-natal and paranatal factors in development of childhood reading disorder', *Monog. Soc. Res. Child Devel.*, **24** (4 Whole No. 73).

KEELEY, K. (1962). 'Pre-natal influence on behaviour of offspring of crowded mice', *Science*, **135**, 44.

KELLY, J. V. (1962). 'Effect of fear upon uterine motility', *Am. J. Obstet. Gynec.*, **83**, 576.

KING, F. J., BOWMAN, B. H., and MORELAND, H. J. (1961). 'Some intellectual correlates of biochemical variability', *Behav. Sci.*, **6**, 297.

KNOBEL, M. (1967). *Psychotherapy and Psychosomatics*, **15(1)**, 34.

KRECH, D., ROSENZWEIG, M. R., and BENNETT, E. L. (1960). *J. Comp. Physiol. Psychol.*, **53**, 509.

KRON, R. E., STEIN, M., and GODDARD, K. E. (1966). 'Newborn sucking behaviour affected by obstetric sedation', *Pediatrics*, **37**, 1012.

LEVINE, S. (1967). 'Maternal and environmental influences on adreno-cortical response to stress in weanling rats', *Science*, **156**, 258.

——, and MULLINS, R. F. (1966). 'Hormonal influences on brain organization in infant rats', *Science*, **152**, 1585.

LIDDICOAT, R. (1968). 'Effects of maternal antenatal decompression treatment on infant mental development', *S. Afr. Med. J.*, **42**, 203.

LIPSITT, L. P. (1969). 'Learning capacities of the human infant', ed. Robinson, R. J. *Brain and Early Behaviour*, 227 (London and New York: Academic Press).

MCDONALD, R. L. (1968). 'The role of emotional factors in obstetric complications: a review', *Psychosom. Med.*, **30**, 222.

MCILWAIN, H. (1966). *Biochemistry and the Central Nervous System* (J. and A. Churchill).

—— (1970). 'Metabolic adaptation in the brain', *Nature*, **226**, 803.

MEIER, G. W., BUNCH, M. E., NOLAN, C. Y., and SCHEIDLER, C. A. (1960). 'Anoxia, behavioural development and learning ability', *Psychol. Monogr.*, **74**, 1 (Whole No. 488).

MONEY, J., and EHRHARDT, A. A. (1968). In ed. Michael, R. *Endocrinology and Human Behaviour*, 32 (London: Oxford University Press).

MORRA, M. (1965). 'Pre-natal sound stimulation on post-natal offspring open-field behavior', *Psychol. Rec.*, **15(4)**, 571.

MURDOCH, B. D. (1968). 'Effects of pre-natal maternal decompression on EEG development of three-year-old children', *S. Afr. Med. J.*, **42**, 1067.

ORME, J. E. (1965). 'Ability and season of birth', *Br. J. Psychol.*, **56(4)**, 471.

PASAMANICK, B., and KNOBLOCH, H. (1966). 'Retrospective studies on epidemiology of reproductive causality', *Merrill-Palmer Quart.*, **12(1)**, 7.

——, and LILIENFELD, A. M. (1955). 'Association of maternal and fetal factors with development of mental deficiency. 1. Abnormalities in pre-natal and paranatal periods', *J. Am. Med. Ass.*, **159**, 155.

——, ROGERS, M. E., and LILIENFELD, A. M. (1956). 'Pregnancy experience and the development of behaviour disorder in children', *Am. J. Psychiat.*, **112**, 613.

PETRE-QUADENS, O., HARDY, J. L., and LEE, C. DE (1969). 'Comparative study of sleep in pregnancy and in the newborn', ed. Robinson, R. J., *Brain and Early Behaviour*, 177 (London and New York: Academic Press).

PRECHTL, H. F. R. (1969). 'Brain and behavioural mechanisms in the human newborn infant', ed. Robinson, R. J., *Brain and Early Behaviour*, 115 (London and New York: Academic Press).

RESSLER, R. H. (1966). 'Inherited environmental influences on the operant behaviour of mice', *J. comp. physiol. Psychol.*, **61**, 264.

RICHARDS, I. D. G. (1969). 'Congenital malformations and environmental influences in pregnancy', *Br. J. prev. soc. Med.*, **23**, 218.

Richards, T. W., and Newberry, H. (1938). 'Studies in fetal behavior; III. Can performance on test items at 6 months postnatally be predicted on the basis of fetal activity?', *Child Devel.*, **9**, 79.
——, ——, and Falgetter, R. (1938). 'Studies in fetal behavior; II. Activity of the human fetus in utero and its relation to other pre-natal conditions, particularly the mother's basal metabolic rate'. *Child Devel.*, **9**, 69.
Robinson, N. M., and Robinson, H. B. (1965). 'Follow-up study of children of low birth weight and control children at school age', *Pediatrics*, **35**(**3**), 425.
Salk, L. (1962). 'Mother's heartbeat as an imprinting stimulus', *Trans. N.Y. Acad. Sci.*, **24**, 753.
—— (1968). 'On prevention of schizophrenia', *Diseases of Nervous System*, **29** (5 Suppl.), 11.
Sanders, E. M., Mefferd, R. B., and Bown, O. H. (1960). 'Verbal-quantitative ability and metabolic characteristics of college students', *Educ. Psychol. Measmt.*, **20**, 491.
Schuster, D. H., and Schuster, L. 'Study of stress and sex ratio in humans', *Proc. 77th Annual Conv. APA*, **4** (Pt. 1), 335.
Sechzer, J. A. (1969). 'Memory deficit in monkey's brain damaged by asphyxia neonatorum', *Exptl. Neurol.*, **24**, **4**, 497.
Sheridan, M. D. (1964). 'Final report of a prospective study of children whose mothers had rubella in early pregnancy', *Br. Med. J.*, **2**, 536.
Singer, J. E., Westphal, M., and Niswander, K. (1968). 'Relationship of weight gain during pregnancy to birth weight and infant growth and development in the first year of life', *Obstet. Gynec.*, **31**, 417.
Sontag, L. W. (1941). 'The significance of fetal environmental differences', *Am. J. Obstet. Gynec.*, **42**, 996.
—— (1966). 'Implications of fetal behaviour and environment for adult personalities', *Ann. N.Y. Acad. Sci.*, **134**, **2**, 782.
——, and Wallace, R. F. (1935). 'The effect of cigarette smoking during pregnancy upon the fetal heart rate', *Am. J. Obstet. Gynec.*, **29**, 3.
Spelt, D. K. (1948). 'The conditioning of the human fetus in utero', *J. exp. Psychol.*, **38**, 338.
Stechler, G. (1964). 'Newborn attention as affected by medication during labour', *Science*, **144**, 315.
Sterman, M. B., and Jeannerod, M. (1967). 'Relationship of fetal activity to maternal EEG sleep stage', *Electrocenceph. clin. Neurophysiol.*, **23**, 81.
Stewart, M. A., Pitts, F. N., Craig, A. G., and Dieruf, W. (1966). 'The hyperactive child syndrome', *Am. J. Orthopsychiatry*, **36**, **5**, 861.
Taft, L. T., and Goldfarb, W. (1964). 'Prenatal and perinatal factors in childhood schizophrenia, *Devel. Med. Child Neurol.*, **6**, 32.
Tartakow, I. J. (1965). 'The teratogenicity of maternal rubella', *J. Pediat.*, **66**, 380.
Thomas, A., Chess, S., and Birch, H. G. (1970). 'The origin of personality', *Sci. Amer.*, **223**, **2**, 102.
Timiras, P. S., Vernadakis, A., and Sherwood, N. M. (1968). 'Development and plasticity of the nervous system', ed. Assali, N. S. *The*

Biology of Gestation. Vol. II, *The Fetus and Neonate,* (London and New York: Academic Press).

TUPPER, C., and WEIL, R. J. (1962). 'The problem of spontaneous abortion: IX. The treatment of habitual abortions by psychotherapy', *Am. J. Obstet. Gynec.*, **83**, 421.

VERNON, P. E. (1969). *Intelligence and Cultural Environment* (London: Methuen).

VIERCK, C. J., KING, F. A., and FERM, V. H. (1966). 'Effects of pre-natal hypoxia upon activity and emotionality of the rat', *Psychon. Sci.*, **4**, 87.

WALTERS, C. E. (1965). 'Prediction of post-natal development from fetal activity', *Child Devl.*, **36**(3), 801.

WEHMER, F., PORTER, R. H., and SCALES, B. (1970). 'Pre-mating and pregnancy stress in rats affects behaviour of grandpups', *Nature,* **227**, 622.

WEITZMAN, E. D., and GRAZIANI, L. J. (1968). 'Maturation and topography of auditory evoked response of the prematurely born infant', *Devl. Psychobiol.*, **1**(2), 79.

WIENER, G. (1968). 'Scholastic achievement at age 12–13 of prematurely born infants', *J. Sp. Educ.*, **2**(3), 237.

WIGGLESWORTH, J. S. (1969). 'Malnutrition and brain development', *Devl. Med. Child Neurol.*, **11**, 783.

WILLERMAN, L., and CHURCHILL, J. A. (1967). 'Intelligence and birth weight in identical twins', *Child Devl.*, **38**(3), 623.

WILLIAMS, R. J. (1956). *Biochemical Individuality* (New York: Wiley).

WINDLE, W. F. (1968). 'Brain damage at birth: functional and structural modifications with time', *J. Am. Med. Ass.*, **209**, **9**, 1967.

—— (1969). 'Brain damage by asphyxia at birth', *Sci. Am.*, **221**, **4**, 76.

WOLFF, S. (1967). 'The contribution of obstetric complications to the aetiology of behaviour disorders in childhood', *J. Child Psychol. Psychiat.*, **8**, 51.

WOOLLAM, D. H. M., and MILLEN, J. W. (1960). 'Influence of thyroxine on the incidence of harelip in the "Strong A" line of mice', *Br. med. J.*, **1**, 1253.

YARROW, M. R. (1963). 'Problems of methods in parent-child research', *Child Devl.*, **34**, 215.

YERUSHALMY, J. (1962). 'Statistical considerations and evaluation of epidemiological evidence', eds. James, G., and Rosenthal, T. *Tobacco and Health,* 208 (Springfield, Ill.: C. C. Thomas).

Further reading

JOFFE, J. M. (1969). *Pre-natal Determinants of Behaviour* (Oxford: Pergamon Press).

MONTAGU, M. F. ASHLEY (1962). *Pre-natal Influences* (Sringfield, Ill.: C. C. Thomas).

PASAMANICK, B., and KNOBLOCH, H. (1966). 'Retrospective studies on the epidemiology of reproductive causality', *Merrill-Palmer Quart.*, **12**(1), 7.

SONTAG, L. W. (1966). 'Implications of fetal behavior and environment for adult personalities', *Ann. N.Y. Acad. Sci.* 134, **2**, 72.

APPENDIX 1

Fetal growth charts

Anthropometric Gestation Charts are extremely useful for the rapid assessment of a newborn's rate of fetal growth as well as for the international comparison of results. Remember that these charts are derived from a specific population which may or may not be relevant to your particular hospital.

TECHNIQUE OF MEASUREMENT

Head circumference. Is measured around the largest occipital frontal circumference with a tape-measure exerting gentle pressure.

Crown-heel. Use a board with a fixed head and sliding right-angled foot-piece. The assistant holds the baby's head firmly against the fixed end of the board. The head is held with Frankfort's plane vertically, i.e. an imaginary line from the highest point on the auditory meatus to the lowest point on the margin of the orbit and with the bi-auricular plane horizontally. The examiner presses the baby's knees firmly down over the patella with his left hand (avoid placing one's fingers in the infant's popliteal fossa) and with the right hand, slide the footpiece to contact the baby's feet. One must ensure that the baby is relaxed and his feet are at right angles.

WEIGHT FOR GESTATIONAL AGE TABLES

TABLE 1. *Male, first pregnancies*

Gestation (completed weeks)	*Percentile* 5	10	25	50	75	90	95
32	1·00	1·22	1·55	1·76	2·06	2·41	2·72
33	1·33	1·54	1·85	2·08	2·34	2·68	3·01
34	1·63	1·83	2·12	2·37	2·67	2·92	3·20
35	1·89	2·08	2·37	2·62	2·94	3·19	3·42
36	2·12	2·31	2·58	2·85	3·16	3·43	3·61
37	2·32	2·50	2·76	3·04	3·33	3·62	3·78
38	2·48	2·66	2·91	3·20	3·49	3·76	3·91

Continued overleaf

Weight for Gestational Age Tables—continued

Gestation (completed weeks)	Percentile 5	10	25	50	75	90	95
39	2·61	2·78	3·03	3·32	3·61	3·88	4·03
40	2·71	2·87	3·13	3·42	3·71	3·98	4·14
41	2·77	2·93	3·19	3·48	3·78	4·07	4·22
42	2·80	2·96	3·23	3·51	3·82	4·13	4·27

TABLE 2. *Male, second and subsequent pregnancies*

Gestation (completed weeks)	Percentile 5	10	25	50	75	90	95
32	1·30	1·47	1·75	1·99	2·33	2·65	2·79
33	1·57	1·75	2·03	2·29	2·63	2·94	3·10
34	1·81	2·00	2·28	2·56	2·89	3·18	3·38
35	2·03	2·23	2·51	2·80	3·13	3·43	3·62
36	2·22	2·43	2·70	3·01	3·33	3·64	3·83
37	2·39	2·60	2·87	3·19	3·51	3·82	4·01
38	2·54	2·74	3·02	3·34	3·66	3·97	4·15
39	2·66	2·86	3·13	3·46	3·77	4·09	4·26
40	2·75	2·95	3·22	3·55	3·86	4·17	4·33
41	2·83	3·01	3·28	3·60	3·92	4·23	4·37
42	2·88	3·04	3·31	3·63	3·95	4·25	4·37

TABLE 3. *Female, first pregnancies*

Gestation (completed weeks)	Percentile 5	10	25	50	75	90	95
32	1·05	1·26	1·53	1·83	2·10	2·41	2·71
33	1·33	1·54	1·81	2·11	2·38	2·64	2·92
34	1·58	1·79	2·07	2·35	2·63	2·89	3·10
35	1·81	2·02	2·29	2·58	2·85	3·10	3·30
36	2·01	2·21	2·49	2·77	3·04	3·31	3·46
37	2·19	2·38	2·66	2·94	3·21	3·46	3·59
38	2·34	2·53	2·80	3·08	3·35	3·59	3·71
39	2·47	2·64	2·91	3·19	3·46	3·70	3·82
40	2·57	2·73	3·00	3·27	3·54	3·79	3·93
41	2·65	2·80	3·05	3·33	3·60	3·86	4·02
42	2·70	2·83	3·08	3·36	3·63	3·91	4·03

TABLE 4. *Female, second and subsequent pregnancies*

Gestation (completed weeks)	*Percentile* 5	10	25	50	75	90	95
32	1·22	1·34	1·62	2·00	2·44	2·69	2·78
33	1·49	1·62	1·91	2·26	2·68	2·94	3·06
34	1·73	1·88	2·17	2·50	2·89	3·17	3·31
35	1·95	2·11	2·40	2·71	3·08	3·37	3·53
36	2·14	2·31	2·59	2·90	3·24	3·54	3·72
37	2·30	2·48	2·76	3·06	3·39	3·69	3·88
38	2·44	2·62	2·90	3·19	3·51	3·82	4·01
39	2·55	2·73	3·00	3·29	3·61	3·92	4·11
40	2·64	2·81	3·08	3·37	3·69	3·99	4·18
41	2·70	2·86	3·13	3·42	3·74	4·04	4·22
42	2·73	2·88	3·14	3·45	3·78	4·07	4·23

THOMSON, A. M., BILLEWICZ, W. Z., and HYTTEN, F. E. (1968). *J. Obstet. Gynaec. Br. Commonw.*, **75**, 903–16.

WEIGHT FOR GESTATIONAL AGE TABLES OF LUBCHENCO

Intrauterine growth as estimated from live born birth weight data at 24–42 weeks of gestation.

TABLE 5. *Male*

Gestational age (weeks)	*Patients (no.)*	*Smoothed percentiles* 10	25	50	75	90
24	13	610	730	830	1,020	1,230
25	12	685	790	880	1,040	1,260
26	43	760	875	965	1,110	1,330
27	38	835	970	1,080	1,215	1,435
28	64	915	1,075	1,205	1,350	1,570
29	80	995	1,180	1,330	1,495	1,720
30	61	1,085	1,290	1,465	1,650	1,875
31	88	1,195	1,415	1,600	1,830	2,050
32	66	1,320	1,550	1,760	2,045	2,280
33	62	1,470	1,710	1,970	2,310	2,575
34	74	1,645	1,920	2,220	2,620	2,920
35	140	1,875	2,180	2,520	2,885	3,190

Continued overleaf

Table 5. Male—contiuned

Gestational age (weeks)	*Patients (no.)*	*Smoothed percentiles* 10	25	50	75	90
36	118	2,105	2,410	2,745	3,090	3,385
37	188	2,330	2,625	2,930	3,245	3,540
38	354	2,505	2,795	3,080	3,380	3,665
39	504	2,630	2,915	3,200	3,505	3,780
40	576	2,700	2,995	3,290	3,610	3,880
41	312	2,735	3,035	3,330	3,670	3,940
42	164	2,730	3,005	3,310	3,660	3,995

Total patients 2,921

TABLE 6. *Female*

Gestational age (weeks)	*Patients (no.)*	*Smoothed percentiles* 10	25	50	75	90
24	11	490	645	760	980	1,250
25	15	600	740	845	1,050	1,295
26	25	700	830	935	1,125	1,350
27	34	790	925	1,035	1,210	1,420
28	54	870	1,020	1,140	1,320	1,530
29	63	945	1,115	1,255	1,455	1,690
30	48	1,025	1,215	1,380	1,600	1,880
31	59	1,125	1,330	1,515	1,760	2,100
32	58	1,250	1,465	1,675	1,970	2,330
33	56	1,400	1,630	1,875	2,275	2,620
34	71	1,550	1,825	2,155	2,555	2,920
35	84	1,730	2,060	2,410	2,795	3,160
36	84	1,960	2,320	2,630	2,980	3,335
37	184	2,220	2,520	2,800	3,120	3,450
38	282	2,405	2,680	2,940	3,235	3,545
39	506	2,540	2,810	3,060	3,340	3,640
40	588	2,630	2,905	3,160	3,440	3,720
41	320	2,660	2,950	3,210	3,520	3,795
42	172	2,630	2,940	3,210	3,550	3,840

Total patients 2,714

LUBCHENCO, L. O., HANSMAN, C., DRESSLER, M., and BOYD, E. (1963). *Paediatrics*, **32**, 793–80.

CROWN–HEEL LENGTH

Intrauterine growth in length as estimated from live births at gestational ages from 26–42 weeks.

TABLE 7.

Gestational age (week)	*Patients (no.)*	*Mean*	*Smoothed percentiles (cm) both sexes* 10	25	50	75	90
26	30	36·5	30·8	32·9	35·5	37·5	39·9
27	21	37·0	31·8	34·1	36·6	38·6	41·0
28	46	38·5	33·0	35·5	37·8	39·8	42·2
29	53	39·0	34·4	36·8	39·0	40·9	43·1
30	47	40·5	36·1	38·3	40·3	42·2	44·5
31	54	41·4	37·5	39·7	41·6	43·5	45·9
32	62	43·5	38·8	41·1	43·2	45·0	47·2
33	69	44·8	39·9	42·3	44·7	46·2	48·4
34	111	45·2	41·0	43·4	45·8	47·3	49·4
35	149	46·8	42·0	44·6	46·7	48·1	50·2
36	189	47·5	43·1	45·6	47·4	48·8	50·9
37	345	47·8	44·1	46·5	48·0	49·3	51·3
38	595	48·5	44·9	47·1	48·4	49·8	51·7
39	957	48·9	45·5	47·6	48·8	50·1	52·0
40	1,084	49·4	45·8	47·9	49·2	50·5	52·3
41	589	49·6	46·0	48·1	49·5	50·8	52·6
42	315	49·8	46·2	48·2	49·7	51·0	52·8

Total patients 4,716

LUBCHENCO, L. O., HANSMAN, C., and BOYD, E. (1968). *Paediatrics*, **37**, 403–8.

OCCIPITAL FRONTAL CIRCUMFERENCE

Intrauterine growth in head circumference (O.F.C.) as estimated from live births at gestational ages from 26–42 weeks.

TABLE 8.

Gestational age (week)	*Patients (no.)*	*Mean*	*Smoothed percentiles (cm) both sexes* 10	25	50	75	90
26	24	26·1	22·4	23·6	25·2	26·6	28·5
27	20	26·1	23·2	24·4	25·8	27·2	28·9
28	40	26·9	24·3	25·4	26·7	28·0	29·4
29	49	27·9	25·3	26·4	27·6	28·8	30·2

Continued overleaf

Table 8.—continued

Gestational age (week)	*Patients (no.)*	*Mean*	*Smoothed percentiles (cm) both sexes* 10	25	50	75	90
30	49	28·9	26·2	27·4	28·6	29·7	31·1
31	53	29·8	26·9	28·2	29·6	30·5	31·9
32	58	30·1	27·6	29·0	30·4	31·4	32·7
33	65	31·5	28·4	29·8	31·2	32·1	33·4
34	103	31·9	29·2	30·6	31·9	32·9	34·0
35	149	32·4	30·0	31·3	32·5	33·4	34·5
36	186	32·9	30·6	31·8	32·9	33·8	34·9
37	353	33·2	31·1	32·3	33·2	34·1	35·2
38	611	33·4	31·4	32·5	33·4	34·3	35·4
39	961	33·6	31·6	32·8	33·7	34·6	35·7
40	1,097	33·8	31·8	33·0	34·0	34·8	35·9
41	587	34·1	32·0	33·2	34·2	35·0	36·0
42	315	34·2	32·1	33·4	34·3	35·1	36·2

Total patients 4,720

LUBCHENCO, L. O., HANSMAN, C., and BOYD, E. (1968). *Paediatrics*, **37**, 403–8.

ADDITIONAL ANTHROPOMETRIC TABLES

Usher and McLean described tables measuring weight, length (crown–heel), foot length, head, chest, abdominal, thigh circumference, and double skin fold thickness.

USHER, R., and MCLEAN, F. (1969). *J. Pediat.*, **74**, 901–10.

Kitchen, W. H., described the relationship between birth weight and gestational age in an Australian hospital population.

Aust. Pediat. J. (1968), **4**, 29–37.

Head circumference, length and placental weight of infants in an Australian population.

Aust. Pediat. J. (1968), **4**, 105–9.

ASSESSMENT OF GESTATIONAL AGE

From the various methods of assessing gestational age, e.g. neurological examinations, X-ray and nerve conduction, the method utilizing external characteristics has been selected.

List of definitions

Skin colour. Estimated by inspection when the infant is quiet, and not shortly after crying.

0 = Dark red.
1 = Uniformly pink.
2 = Pale pink, though the colour may vary over different parts of the body – i.e., some parts may be very pale.
3 = Pale; nowhere really pink, except on the ears, lips, palms and soles.

Skin opacity. Estimated by inspection of the trunk.

0 = Numerous veins, tributaries, and venules seen clearly, particularly over the abdomen.
1 = Veins and tributaries seen.
2 = A few large blood-vessels seen clearly over the abdomen.
3 = A few large blood-vessels seen indistinctly over the abdomen.
4 = No blood-vessels seen.

Skin texture. Tested by picking up a fold of abdominal skin between finger and thumb, and by inspection.

0 = Very thin, with a gelatinous feel.
1 = Thin and smooth.
2 = Smooth and of medium thickness; irritation, rash and superficial peeling may be present.
3 = Slight thickening and stiff feeling, with superficial cracking and peeling, especially evident on the hands and feet.
4 = Thick and parchment-like, with superficial or deep cracking.

Nipple formation. Estimated by inspection.

0 = Nipple barely visible; no areola.
1 = Nipple well-defined; areola present but not raised.
2 = Nipple well-defined; edge of the areola raised above the skin.

Breast size. Measured by picking up the breast tissue between finger and thumb.

0 = No breast tissue palpable.
1 = Breast tissue palpable on one or both sides, neither being more than 0·5 cm in diameter.
2 = Breast tissue palpable on both sides, one or both being 0·5 to 1 cm in diameter.
3 = Breast tissue palpable on both sides, one or both being more than 1 cm in diameter.

Skull hardness. Estimated by palpation, and by alternate pressure with the first and middle fingers, along the edges of the sutures.

0 = Skull bones feel soft to at least 1 inch from the anterior fontanelle, with only moderate resistance to pressure.
1 = Skull bones appear springy along the edges of the fontanelle, while the centres of the bones feel hard.
2 = Some bones hard, others springy, along the edge of the fontanelle.
3 = Bones hard up to the sutures, but can be displaced easily with gentle pressure.
4 = Bones hard, and cannot be readily displaced with gentle pressure.

Ear form. Assessed by inspection of the upper part of the pinna, above the external meatus.

0 = Almost flat and shapeless pinna, with little or no incurving of the edge.
1 = Incurving of any degree of part of the periphery of the pinna.
2 = Partial incurving of the whole of the upper pinna.
3 = Well-defined incurving of the whole of the upper pinna.

Ear firmness. Tested by palpation and folding of the upper pinna between finger and thumb.

0 = Pinna feels soft, and is easily folded into bizarre positions without springing back into position spontaneously.
1 = Pinna feels soft along the edge and is easily folded, but returns slowly to the correct position spontaneously.
2 = Cartilage can be felt to the edge of the pinna, though it is thin in places, and the pinna springs back readily after being folded.
3 = Pinna firm, with definite cartilage extending to the periphery, and springs back into position immediately after being folded.

Males

0 = Neither testis in the scrotum.
½ = At least one testis low in the inguinal canal, so that it can be drawn into the upper scrotum.
1 = At least one testis high in the scrotum, though it may be drawn into the lowest position.
2 = At least one testis completely descended into the lower scrotum.

Females. Examined with lower limbs half abducted.

0 = Labia majora widely separated, with comparatively large labia minora protruding.
1 = Labia majora almost cover labia minora.
2 = Labia majora cover labia minora completely.

(The half score for grading of the male genitalia is intended to keep the scoring for the two sexes the same, i.e. from 0 to 2.)

Oedema. Tested by inspection and by finger pressure over the tibia for 5 seconds.

0 = Obvious oedema of the feet and hands, with moderate pitting over the tibia.
1 = No obvious oedema, but definite palpable pitting over the tibia.
2 = No oedema detected.

Plantar skin creases. Assessed by noting the creases which persist when the skin of the sole is stretched from toes to heel.

0 = No skin creases present.
1 = Skin creases are faint red marks over the anterior half of the sole.
2 = Creases are definite red marks over more than the anterior half of the sole, and indentation is present over no more than the anterior third.
3 = As (2) but the indentation is present over more than a third of the sole.
4 = Definite deep indentation present over more than the anterior third of the sole.

Lanugo. Examined over the back, holding the infant up to the light.

0 = No lanugo, or very scanty short hairs present.
1 = Abundant, long and thick over the whole back.
2 = Lanugo thinning, especially over the lower back.
3 = Smaller amounts of lanugo, with areas of baldness.
4 = At least half of the back devoid of lanugo.

TABLE 9. *Conversion of total maturity score to predicted gestational age*

Score	*Gestational age (weeks)*	*Score*	*Gestational age (weeks)*	*Score*	*Gestational age (weeks)*
5	28·1	15	35·9	25	40·3
6	29·0	16	36·5	26	40·6
7	29·9	17	37·1	27	40·8
8	30·8	18	37·6	28	41·0
9	31·6	19	38·1	29	41·1
10	32·4	20	38·5	30	41·2
11	33·2	21	39·0	31	41·3
12	33·9	22	39·4	32	41·4
13	34·6	23	39·7	33	41·4
14	35·3	24	40·0	34	41·4

FARR, V., MITCHELL, R. G., NELIGAN, G. A., and PARKIN, J. M. (1966). *Devl. Med. Child Neurol.*, **8**, 507–11.

APPENDIX 2

Technique of amniocentesis

INDICATIONS

Diagnostic

1. Rhesus iso-immunization.
2. Estimation of fetal maturity, cytological, biochemical, radiological.
3. Fetal abnormalities, chromosomal, biochemical, radiological.

Therapeutic

1. Severe hydramnios.
2. Induction of abortion.

TECHNIQUE

Amniocentesis is safely carried out as an out-patient procedure. Having emptied her bladder, the patient lies supine, and the site for puncture is chosen. Abdominal palpation is carefully performed and if the limbs are easily felt, it is unlikely that an anterior placenta is present. Amniocentesis is best performed between the fetal limbs, where there is usually a pool of liquor. If an anterior placenta is suspected the flanks provide alternative sites, especially into the liquor behind the fetal occiput.

Using strict aseptic precautions, including skin preparation, and abdominal towels, about 2 ml of half per cent lignocaine are infiltrated into the skin at the puncture site using a fine needle. There is no need to infiltrate below the skin. After a suitable interval, a spinal needle is passed through the abdominal and uterine walls into the amniotic cavity. The stilette is removed and, using a 20 ml syringe, liquor amnii is aspirated. A pudendal needle can also be used but this probably causes more trauma (as there is no stilette). A firm push is required to pass through the tissues. If pure blood is initially aspirated, suggestive that the placenta has been encountered, further advancement of the needle into the amniotic cavity is necessary.

If this is not successful, another site should be found, rather than 'puddle' in the placenta. If liquor is not obtained, slight alteration of the needle position in the up-and-down direction is usually successful.

When sufficient sample has been taken, the stilette is replaced, and the needle quickly removed. The puncture site is covered with a small circular adhesive plaster. If the fetal heart rate remains satisfactory during the following fifteen minutes, the patient is allowed up.

COMPLICATIONS

There is remarkably little morbidity to either mother or fetus from this procedure. Despite this, the clinician must be certain that the risks from the problem he is investigating outweigh those from amniocentesis.

Blood (originating from the placenta or the myometrium) may contaminate the fluid and interfere with the laboratory test being applied. Bloody taps may occur in up to 5 per cent of cases. Although rare, massive increases in antibody titres have been described in cases of Rhesus iso-immunization, with worsening of the haemolytic disease. Feto-maternal leaks can be detected using the Kleihauer technique. If an anterior placenta is suspected its position can be investigated using simple ultrasonic apparatus (e.g. Doptone or Sonicaid). Placental separation is caused exceedingly rarely.

Occasionally dry taps occur, particularly when the amount of liquor is diminished.

Fetal damage is exceptional. Needling can occur, but it is generally harmless. It must be remembered that rupture of a large cord vessel will result in fetal death, but, happily, it is an unusual complication.

Premature labour is uncommon. Intrauterine infection is rarely encountered.

INDEX